HAPPY MOM
HAPPY KID

Copyright © 2021 Zelmira Crespi and Maria Montt

All rights reserved. No part of this publication may be reproduced, distributed, or transmitted in any form or by any means, including photocopying, recording, or other electronic or mechanical methods, without the prior written permission of the publisher, except in the case of brief quotations embodied in critical reviews and certain other noncommercial uses permitted by copyright law. For permission requests, write to the publisher, addressed "Attention: Permissions Coordinator," at the address below.

Contact information for Zelquin LLC– info@happymomhappykid.com

ISBN: 978-1-7366876-0-4 (print)
ISBN: 978-1-7366876-1-1 (ebook)

Ordering Information:
Special discounts are available on quantity purchases by corporations, associations, and others. For details, contact info@happymomhappykid.com

HAPPY MOM HAPPY KID

A STUDY ON LIFE SATISFACTION IN WOMEN AND HOW TO RECONNECT WITH THE BEST VERSION OF YOU FOR YOUR KIDS

ZELMIRA CRESPI
MARIA LUISA MONTT

Table of Contents

Introduction: The Unspoken Truth 1

Chapter 1: The Rubik's Cube of Motherhood 9

Chapter 2: Labor Day 17

Chapter 3: Identity Collision 23

Chapter 4: Mom Shaming 33

Chapter 5: Going All-In 49

Chapter 6: The Happy Moms Study 63

Chapter 7: Family 101 71

Chapter 8: Friends 87

Chapter 9: Finding Purpose in Work 97

Chapter 10: Your Personal Health Coach for Free 111

Chapter 11: Mental Wellness Is a Priority 123

Chapter 12: Let's Get Going 135

Introduction: The Unspoken Truth

You've probably heard the saying "Happy wife, happy life." In this book, we want to talk about our go-to motto, the concept of "Happy mom, happy kid." We realized that every major bookstore on the planet has shelves and shelves of books claiming to offer the secret to raising kids who are happy, confident, and successful. As moms, we are conditioned from day one to focus on the needs of our families because motherhood is, after all, a gift, a joy, and the job of a lifetime. But sometimes all those amazing feelings are hard to enjoy when other unexpected feelings of loneliness, fear, anxiety, or simply feeling blue come our way. Are we doing something wrong? Did we read the wrong book on how to raise kids?

While also focusing on the baby about to be born or what pediatrician to go to, we women are going through a lot of changes—not only in our bodies, but also emotionally and mentally. So the question is, what about the women behind the moms? Our personal experiences combined with the hard questions we've asked our friends and peers have made us realize that being a mom is not so easy and not so pretty for most of us. Whether we talk about it or not, or allow ourselves to see it, it takes a lot of hard work to pull off motherhood. And with hard work comes hard times. No matter how happy we are to do it, we must acknowledge this.

We've also learned most moms are not OK with expressing the hardships we go through as a whole. We're quick to say that we had a rough night, but we're not quick to realize the amount of massive responsibility that has been placed in our hands, the process it takes to really understand how we're going to navigate it—and how we feel about it—and worst of all, how we tend to stay quiet when we might need a helping hand in all of this. For years we had been talking about this huge change of pace that motherhood brings, but we had never really been able to define it until now.

HEY THERE! CALL ME Z

I'm a communication specialist, writer, and dark humor professional. I relocated to Miami in 2010. It wasn't too difficult of a transition for me since I had lived abroad my entire life. My father was a United Nations representative for the Development Program, and we lived in the US, Panama, the Dominican Republic, Argentina, Paraguay, and Spain. All of my family was born and raised in Uruguay. Uruguay is mostly known for soccer (first ever World Cup destination); extensive green pastures where our coveted grass-fed cattle roam freely; and long, amazing beaches. Our life abroad was a great experience that gave me a good perspective to observe life's changes and processes, adapt to the different, and welcome changes in my life constantly. Motherhood was a bit of a pickle to adapt to, though. More on this later.

HI, EVERYONE! I'M M

I have a bachelor's degree in child psychology and a career in online marketing. I'm a bit of a sour patch; I can be blunt and direct but sweet at the same time. When I moved to Miami in 2010, it was the first time I had ever lived outside of my home country of Chile. To top it off, I had an eight-month-old baby and another on the way! Chile is well known for its wines that go great with Z's country's red meat and the Andes mountains (not the chocolate).

We're both hard workers, love our families, love being moms, and love our lives. When we get together, our conversations run around the topics of women's empowerment, using our talents and time as best as possible, and applying our know-how to get through challenges in life, love, and work. We're both passionate about whatever it is that we do and always take our ups and downs like the best life lessons we could have. This is what has made us stick together as friends all these years.

Long story short, one morning we found ourselves with a book project that we somehow both desperately needed to get done. We realized that, for quite some time, we had both felt a need to really talk about, investigate, and share *what the hell happens to us once we become mothers*. Very often we find ourselves with groups of moms talking for hours about what our kids do right or wrong, discussing what our plans are for them, and comparing notes on each other's experiences and the kids' milestones. At the end of the day, every mom wants and needs to see that her child is doing well, that we are managing their lives in the best way possible. But we've come to the realization that in order for our children to be happy, they need us moms to be happy first.

HELLO MATRESCENCE

Emerging research reveals that the onset of motherhood often plunges women into a severe identity crisis known as *matrescence*. This period is experienced to some extent by *100 percent of new moms* as they struggle to redefine themselves in a complex new role.[1]

The term matrescence was first coined in 1975 by medical anthropologist Dana Raphael, as a combination of the words "maternal" and "adolescence."[2] Just as the teenage years are the time of life when we become adults, matrescence is the time when we become mothers. Both processes are complicated, stressful, and drawn out.

Psychiatrist Daniel Stern, a well-known expert researcher in the field of early affective mother-child bonding, says in the book *The Birth of a Mother* that creating another human is only part of what it takes to become a mom.[3] He wrote that new mothers also have to create a new identity for themselves, and that can be just as difficult as making the baby. According to Dr. Stern, becoming a mother is one of the biggest *physical* changes a woman can undergo, as well as one of the biggest *psychological* and *emotional* changes.[4]

> *"In my pregnancy and through becoming a mother, I lost a lot of myself. And I've struggled, and I still do struggle being a mom. It's really hard."*
>
> —*Adele*, acceptance speech, 59th Annual Grammy Awards

---

1 Alexandra Sacks, "Matrescence: The Developmental Transition to Motherhood," Psychology Today (Sussex Publishers, April 8, 2019), https://www.psychologytoday.com/us/blog/motherhood-unfiltered/201904/matrescence-the-developmental-transition-motherhood.
2 Dana Raphael, *Being Female: Reproduction, Power, and Change* (The Hague: Mouton Publishers, 1975), 65.
3 Daniel N. Stern et al., *The Birth of a Mother: How the Motherhood Experience Changes You Forever* (New York: Basic Books, 1998).
4 Stern et al., *The Birth of a Mother*.

If we look deeper into the hard parts of learning to be a new mom, we see the winding road we all know is there. If we have our baby at a hospital, for example, the staff makes us complete a questionnaire that asks if we feel a bit "off." This is to evaluate if we have postpartum depression (PPD), which is a deep, dark depression and a hard reality that hits one in every seven new moms. It's the first time we are met with, "Are you sure you're OK?" after giving birth, and it might just be our last. Once we've confirmed we don't have PPD, then we are expected to experience a bit of baby blues at the most, but that's pretty much it.

What Alexandra Sacks, MD, reproductive psychiatrist, realized was that she treated a lot of new moms worrying that they were suffering from postpartum depression simply because they were not having all of the positive emotions they were told, shown, or advised they would and should have. She says that "[t]he process of becoming a mother, which anthropologists call 'matrescence,' has been largely unexplored in the medical community. Instead of focusing on the woman's identity transition, more research is focused on how the baby turns out. But a woman's story, in addition to how her psychology impacts her parenting, is important to examine, too."[5]

We have always been a bit alarmed about how little people talk about how one truly feels during the process of becoming a mom, turning it into an unspoken truth. But every time we signed that paper, all four times we each delivered babies, we were quick to answer no, all the while knowing that the answer wasn't so black and white and that it could change eventually. Matrescence answers the question of what happens in that big gap between the super heavy postpartum reality and the easy, breezy perfect mom fantasy.

The first time we heard the word matrescence, it was like opening the door of a room that nobody knew was there. But once we peeked in, we found lots of familiar stuff inside—the physical pain of breastfeeding for some; for others, the crying toddler desperate for our attention while we change the new baby; losing our nightly 8 p.m. chat with our partner because we hit the bed like a rock; the strange sensation of being stuck while everybody else goes on with their lives; the complicated decision to go back to work part time or full time; childcare; guilt; and so on. Motherhood

---

5 Alexandra Sacks, "The Birth of a Mother," *New York Times*, May 8, 2017, https://www.nytimes.com/2017/05/08/well/family/the-birth-of-a-mother.html.

is amazing in many ways and also one of the hardest things we might go through without any sort of preparation.

When we first became moms, we quickly realized there were a few facts we'd failed to grasp about how we would be expected to behave now that we had babies. We weren't prepared for how quickly everything would change. Some new moms are lucky enough to have a friend or close relative that can catch them up on the new rules of the world they are walking into. Others might receive a gentle warning from the nurse at the hospital. But nothing can really prepare us for motherhood until we experience it for ourselves. It's a massive shift, inside and out.

A WEEK'S WORTH OF CHICKEN AND RICE, BY M

I can still remember the exact moment when I opened the front door to my small two-bedroom apartment and found my friend with a priceless gift in her hands. I had bags under my eyes, a week-old baby in my arms, and a one-year-old clinging to my legs. I was exhausted, and the last thing I wanted was a house visit of any kind. Survival mode was on and real.

"I didn't know what to get you so I thought maybe this could be helpful," she said as she handed me a huge aluminum tray half-filled with rice and half-filled with cooked chicken. I softly chuckled, said "thanks," and closed the door. That would turn out to be our meals for the rest of the week.

I still remember it to this day as the least-expected gift, but the most valued one. I had no idea how tired I could feel, so much so that I could barely get myself to cook my own chicken and rice meal. So, chicken and rice it was, and eventually I started to feel a bit better, had more energy, and got back to cooking basics.

HELLO, IS IT ME YOU'RE LOOKING FOR? BY Z

One muggy August afternoon, I showed up at M's house holding a struggling toddler from each hand. This particular day, I was exhausted and plain ol' bored!

"I need to do something with my life," I said as we slumped down onto the couches in M's living room. "I don't know where I went, but I need to get back to me." I continued, "How did I get here? Why am I not at an office like I

always planned to be as a mom? Why do I drive a minivan when I swore—SWORE, Maria—that I would NEVER drive a minivan. What happened to me?? Where did I go?"

I had become a stay-at-home mom soon after my first child, Josefina, was born with a heart condition and Down syndrome. Rather than hiring a team for round-the-clock care, I talked it over with my husband, and we opted for me to stay at home until our daughter was old enough to start school. "Josefina needs *me*," I reasoned.

By the time I walked into M's house that day, I had two kids, and my plans to go back to work and take on personal projects were nowhere in sight. I was grateful to have been able to stay home with Josefina, but now that I was officially a mom of two, I realized that I needed some me time. For me, that meant finding something that made me use my talents and capacity outside of the home and, of course, making my own money! As I'd always said, I was brought up to be a professional, independent woman. Staying at home, dedicated to kids and housework with no reimbursement, got to be a big burden, and I didn't know how to handle it!

This was it. The problem so many moms—maybe *every* mom—goes through: a loss of self. In fact, it's impossible to become a mom without surrendering some of ourselves in the process.

But why does this happen, can we fix it, and how does this change affect our level of happiness and overall satisfaction in life? We decided to find out. The two of us teamed up with another friend, who is an academic psychologist, to conduct a study in which we surveyed over 600 women. If all women go through this self-redefinition once we become mothers, why do some seem to thrive in their lives after becoming moms and others feel stuck or without any life purpose? We wanted to identify the tools that moms can use to give ourselves the satisfaction we need to keep us healthy, positive, and moving forward in our best way possible.

We discovered that it's possible for us moms to successfully redefine ourselves through life, be grateful, love our families, not regret anything, *and still* want more at the same time.

In this book, we'll show you the following:

- Where that strange sensation of *feeling off* or having *brain fog* as a mother comes from.

INTRODUCTION: THE UNSPOKEN TRUTH

- How guilt, shame, and unrealistic expectations are robbing us of joy—and how to stop the cycle.
- How even though some feelings that aren't severe enough to be postpartum depression are still important enough to address.
- How we gradually become the second priority in our own lives and how it can be tricky to get back to taking care of ourselves.
- What moms can learn from poker players.
- Where our cultural beliefs about motherhood come from.

But first, we need to explain why motherhood is like a Rubik's Cube.

CHAPTER 1

The Rubik's Cube of Motherhood

You hear that your heart doubles in size the day you become a mom (and it's 100 percent true, by the way). But you don't hear about how your identity also shifts the moment you give birth, and how this shift can leave you scrambling to reinvent yourself in your new role. You also hear that you'll never love anyone else as much as you love your own children (and that's definitely true), but you don't hear about how frustrated you'll be when your kids spill things, don't do as they're told, or you burn dinner again while bathing someone for the third time that day, for example. And, of course, you hear you'll never regret becoming a mom (true again), but you don't hear about the days when you look with envy at photos on social media of your childless friends.

Think back to before you became a mom—back to when you were building an identity for yourself. Those were the days when you had confidence about who you were, where you were going, and what you wanted out of life. You worked hard on yourself, your career, and your education. You took care of your own needs. Then pregnancy came around, and as soon as you saw that little red stripe on the pregnancy test, your mom identity struggle began.

Matrescence has been described by psychologists and mental health professionals for decades, including Grete L. Bibring, the first female full clinical professor at Harvard Medical School.[6] Bibring did extensive research on women during and after pregnancy, studying their psychological needs and processes. An article titled "A Study of the Psychological Processes in Pregnancy and of the Earliest Mother-Child Relationship," by Bibring and colleagues, states, "Pregnancy, like puberty or menopause, is regarded as a period of crisis involving profound endocrine and general somatic as well as psychological changes. The crisis of pregnancy is basically a normal occurrence and indeed even essential part of growth, which must precede and prepare maturational integration."[7] This means that the hormonal, body, and mental movement that we women go through during pregnancy is so strong that we have to check in with ourselves and see how we're feeling. Also, it shows that we're living with a real reason for thinking that some things might have shifted out of place.

Nearly every mom feels a loss of identity at some point; it's an almost universal experience. Many women get so caught up in becoming a mom that we completely lose ourselves in the glory of motherhood. Getting a firm sense of control over who we are as a mom turns out to be a bit more complicated than most of us expect.

We have nicknamed this the "Rubik's Cube challenge" after the famous multicolored plastic puzzle boxes developed in 1974 by Hungarian architecture professor Erno Rubik.[8] Rubik invented the cube while he was teaching a class on descriptive geometry. He saw its potential and went on to patent it as a toy, which most of us have had the pleasure of trying to figure out time and time again.

What makes the Rubik's Cube so addictive is that, at first glance, it seems like it should be simple to solve—but it's not. In many ways, the cube is just like matrescence. Imagine that the little squares on the Rubik's Cube represent your tastes, feelings, dreams, and personality traits. Every time you enter a new phase of life, the colors get shuffled around, and it takes you some time to learn the new moves to get things organized in a way

---

6 "Grete L. Bibring: The Modern Woman," Center for History of Medicine at Countway Library, accessed October 7, 2020, https://collections.countway.harvard.edu/onview/exhibits/show/grete-bibring-the-modern-woman.
7 G. L. Bibring et al., "A study of the psychological processes in pregnancy and of the earliest mother-child relationship," *The Psychoanalytic Study of the Child* 16, no. 1 (1961): 9–72.
8 Alexandra Alter, "He Invented the Rubik's Cube. He's Still Learning from It," *New York Times*, September 16, 2020, https://www.nytimes.com/2020/09/16/books/erno-rubik-rubiks-cube-inventor-cubed.html.

that feels comfortable to you. But once you learn how it works, everything starts to line up for you effortlessly.

You might have experienced the Rubik's Cube challenge as a child when you had to move on to middle school just as you were really starting to get the hang of elementary school. It commonly strikes during the teenage years when it can feel like adulthood is coming on just when you were getting childhood figured out. When the Rubik's Cube challenge strikes, it feels like all of those colorful squares you spent years lining up are migrating out of place again.

This process specifically happens when women become moms; you experience a slow and silent process of feeling like you're fading away from the woman you used to be before you had kids. You might start to lose track of your old interests and your passions without even realizing it. Your Rubik's Cube is shuffling itself up. When you get the hang of your baby crawling, the baby will start to walk. And just as you get the diapers under control, it'll be time for potty training. For many moms, the Rubik's Cube challenge can be exhausting. The good news is that there is a way to stop yourself from getting lost in the process as you go through motherhood.

GOODBYE, SASHIMI, AND HELLO, PANKO-BREADED SHRIMP, BY Z

I walked into a dinner party with my friends a few months after becoming pregnant with my first child. I had on my power suit with my black maternity pants from The Gap, and I was feeling like I had this preggo thing down to a T. We all sat down, ordered, and started chatting about life.

Then dinner arrived. Everyone else had already received their plate. When the waitress put down my plate of sashimi, a friend leaned over with concern on her face and asked softly, "Um...are you sure you can eat that?" I looked at the raw seafood I so desperately wanted to chomp down on after a long day at the office and realized, suddenly, "No, I can't." I was clearly caught off guard. It's common knowledge that pregnant women aren't supposed to eat raw fish, but this was the first time it had applied to me!

The vomiting from the first four months had finally stopped, and I was feeling much better. But somewhere in the midst of being at the office all day, sitting down with my good friends, and talking about anything and everything, I had lost track of the fact that I was still pregnant. I thought, "If I forgot about this, does this mean I'll forget about more important things later when the baby is born?" I began to worry if I would be able to adapt to all of this or if I would fail. My cube had shifted without me even noticing.

"Should I call my doctor and ask?" I thought, knowing that this did not qualify as an emergency phone call. I sighed and started to analyze the sushi menu, trying to find something—anything—that was not raw. Offering my amazing sashimi platter to my already full friends, I waved to the waitress, asking if there were any better options than the chicken teriyaki. What was obvious before, I realized, was no longer clear. I now had to start over and learn the ways of a pregnant woman because now that was me.

My Rubik's Cube was shifting—fast.

Some extra perceptive mothers notice this gradual shift as it is happening. Others just wake up one morning and see it all of a sudden. There are also those moms who continue going about their usual business, oblivious, until they accidentally try to do something that's no longer allowed and get slapped on the wrist (like Z with her sashimi).

Little by little you embrace the vomiting, the swollen ankles, the hot flashes, the decaf coffee, the prenatal vitamins (aka horse pills), the peeing *all* the time, and the strangers rubbing your belly as if it were a lamp with a genie in it. You aren't necessarily thrilled with all of these changes (especially the belly rubbing), but you bear them all because you're confident that the end result is going to be the best and most rewarding thing in the entire world: motherhood. You do it gladly, without question. But this shift does have a very real effect on your identity.

Another thing complicates the matter: the expectation that every mother-to-be will always be warm, happy, and *so excited*. After all, simply by nature of just being pregnant, you are virtuous. If you get cranky or snap at anyone (although you tried your hardest not to), you might be deemed unfit to be a mother. Mothers are patient, after all, and kind. They don't lose their temper. Ever.

Matrescence is subtle, and it starts before you even realize it. Most moms start to notice their identity shift after the baby is born, but it can begin the instant you first realize you are pregnant. This is when your Mom Responsibilities kick in for the first time.

AN ADVIL SUPERHERO, BY M

I was a newlywed on vacation with my husband, and I knew I was supposed to get my period. So, when I started to have some ovary pains, I reached for my trusty Advil, which had taken the pain away so many times before—once a month for the last 10 years. But for some reason, I paused with the pill halfway to my mouth. I turned to my husband and said, "What if I'm pregnant? A pregnant woman can't take Advil, right?"

At the time, I was 24 years old. I didn't know much about the effects of a single Advil on early-stage pregnancy, but I'd heard it was frowned upon. So, I decided I was better safe than sorry, and I skipped the Advil—just in case.

But then the pain started to get worse. A few hours later it was getting to the point where it was unbearable. "Maybe I should take an Advil?" My husband shook his head. In a very loving tone, he proposed that I should "suck it up" until we got back to our house. Once we arrived, the pain continued, but no period came. So, I took my first pregnancy test ever. Sure enough, it was positive.

At that moment, I was so proud of myself for "sucking it up" and not taking that Advil. After all, I had just saved my baby's life! Applause, applause. Cheers to the best new mother out there: moi.

Little did I know that this one decision was the first unseen sign that my Rubik's Cube was beginning to move. I had decided not to take my usual Advil—even though I felt pain—because of the mere chance that someone else might be affected in some way by it in the distant future. Maybe. I had entered matrescence before I even knew I was pregnant.

As soon as you get pregnant, you are no longer able to do many things you want to in your life. Now, suddenly, you have to filter each decision you make through the implications it will have on your kids.

We've made a list of all the little not-so-obvious signs of Rubik's Cube movement during pregnancy—as well as the big, glaring ones you're probably familiar with:

- **Meds:** Medications you normally wouldn't think twice about taking can become dangerous during pregnancy.[9] We don't care how

---

[9] "Pregnant or thinking of getting pregnant?" Centers for Disease Control and Prevention, accessed October 7, 2020, https://www.cdc.gov/pregnancy/meds/treatingfortwo/facts.html.

much snot is coming out of your nose or how puffy your eyes are, you'll just have to deal with it. Be thankful for Tylenol; at least you can take that.[10] If you need anything else, call Grandma, a Chinese herbalist, or your local yoga instructor. Just don't go sitting in a sauna or steam room because you might have a drop in blood pressure and need several people to carry you out to get fresh air. Think smart.

- **Work:** Oh, you have a good job, do you? Aspirations? How nice. So, what are you going to do after maternity leave ends? Are you going to want to go back to work? Really? Get ready to face down an army of individuals who will pummel you incessantly with big existential questions starting the second you get pregnant. It's like someone pays them to keep you as anxious as possible about the future so that you start exercising the internal alarm system all mothers have about returning to work.

- **Food:** You have a well-balanced diet of all of the main food groups. Sure, maybe you take the occasional puff from your friend's cigarette at a dinner party, but overall you're a healthy woman. Now, however, for some inexplicable reason, your brain craves a strict diet of sushi, prosciutto, wine, and mojitos—and you desperately want to smoke like the Marlboro Man. The forbidden fruit effect takes over, and you miss that plump piece of pink raw fish like it's your old boyfriend going off to summer camp when you were 15. Sob.

- **Plans and trips:** Oh, you found great prices on tickets to Hawaii for your next trip with the girlfriends? How fuuuun! Wait, how many months pregnant are you going to be? Oh, that's too bad, Mommy, you'll be nesting in full force by then because your D-day will be too close for travel!

Everything starts to shift once we get pregnant. Again, most of the time we take this on without complaint. It's just part of the process. If we do have any minor misgivings, they are, of course, settled with the great conclusion that "it'll all be worth it." Yet, what we often fail to notice is that our inner self has started to shift, and it's a difficult process. Matrescence has begun even before we've technically become a mom.

---

10 "What Pain Relievers Are Safe During Pregnancy?" WebMD, accessed October 7, 2020, https://www.webmd.com/baby/pain-relievers-that-are-safe-during-pregnancy#1.

We are not here to tell you how to avoid matrescence. It's all part of the plan, and it's great. We just want to show you how to make it through this tumultuous period in your life without losing control of your Rubik's Cube. First, though, we need to look at the official start of matrescence: the birth of your first child.

CHAPTER 2

Labor Day

"When you have a child, you find yourself suddenly alone with a tiny alien without the instructions for use. Around you, life goes on as always: your friends work, your partner shows up only from time to time, your mother or mother in law [sic] either don't show up or are too intrusive. You find yourself living a new experience, a titanic and traumatic one, in utter loneliness; an experience spent in crying, sleepless nights and nappies: it's a madness, at the beginning it's nothing but a mad ride, and you can't share your feelings with anybody."

—Claudia De Lillo, Nonsolomamma blog

Until your first child is born, people will still call you by your real name (you know, the one that's written on your birth certificate). But as soon as that little human pops out of you, it's like your name gets tossed out of the window and is replaced with "Mom." For most mothers, the nurse in the delivery room is the first person to call you the "Mom" word as she hands you your newborn baby.

That's how it was for M.

A MOMMY BREAKDOWN, BY M

My first pregnancy was really fantastic. In fact, I felt so great while I was pregnant that I figured motherhood would be a breeze! I enjoyed my baby bump and felt strong and healthy throughout the entire nine months. The mi-

nor shifts in my Rubik's Cube during pregnancy didn't bother me at all. "This would be a new chapter," I thought. Yes, maybe some things would change but, mostly, I assumed that everything would stay the same as before. I was completely unprepared for matrescence.

The delivery was simple and relatively pain-free. Baby and I were both healthy and happy. Everything looked great. A couple of days later, once all the checkups were taken care of, the doctors sent my new family home. It was, by all accounts, a fabulous birth.

My husband slid into the driver's seat, and I plopped into the back with the baby, with a huge smile on my face. I was happy, excited, and glad to be going home with my new baby. I felt proud and content. We were unquestionably a family now, and this was the real deal. My husband pulled out of the parking lot onto the freeway and we headed home. Then it hit me like a ton of bricks.

Suddenly, I wasn't smiling anymore. I realized there were tears streaming down my face; full-on rivers were pouring down my cheeks and dripping from my chin. I was clearly sobbing, and I just couldn't stop! It was the hardest I have ever cried before or since. It had come completely out of nowhere. My mind began to race.

This was supposed to be the happiest day of my life. I'd just given birth to my first child, and it was a fantastic pregnancy and delivery. Everything had gone awesome. What was wrong with me?

"Is everything…uh…OK?" my husband asked nervously, eyeing me with terror through the rearview mirror. "Should we go back, maybe? To the hospital?"

I shook my head. Everything was going to be alright, I reasoned. I was just having a teeny, tiny internal crisis. No big deal.

At the time, I didn't have the words to describe what was happening to me. But now I do. I had entered full-blown matrescence! I was worried about not being able to take care of my newborn baby and terrified of not knowing who I was anymore. I was suddenly noticing how massively my Rubik's Cube had shifted during the past nine months. And the worst part about it was—nobody had warned me.

This sense of losing part of your former self at the onset of matrescence is far from unique. In fact, many mothers report a feeling of loss right around the birth of their first baby.

No woman is completely prepared to become a mother, either emotionally or mentally. Trying to figure out your new post-mom identity is a massive process of self-discovery. Your previous identity no longer exists, and your whiteboard has been wiped clean. You've suddenly been given a blank slate to create something new.

After you finally do give birth, you are still in control of your own life, but things don't exactly go back to normal. Your body might not seem to snap back to its pre-kid self quite as easily as you'd thought it would. Your desires, motivations, and spontaneous urges might not factor into your decision making as much as they used to. You now have to consider your child's needs before your own every single day. You have to build a new life that revolves around this miniature person. You start to understand why people sometimes say that being a mom is a sacrifice.

> *"If you ask me if I remember what I felt when I realized that something big had changed, I would have to go back to the moment I had my first child. After that, I never really got back to being me again. There is this feeling of wanting to just run away that overwhelms me every once in a while. I have a sense of something heavy pressing on my chest as well when that happens. Sometimes, even anger creeps in, but I'm not really sure about what. Maybe it's because I feel alone, or that I miss my freedom, or I miss being me. I don't know, but it's there and it's real."*
> —*Alexandra,* age 36, mother of three

How is it possible not to know who you are anymore? That's a sign that your Rubik's Cube is shifting. It's scary, but it's necessary and normal. Yes, this is an identity crisis. And, yes, it happens to every mom. Matrescence involves a deep sense of loss because your life has to change in innumerable ways when you give birth to a child.

If you find yourself missing some aspects of your former pre-mom identity, know that you're not alone. We all long for some parts of our old life back. Nostalgia is very real, and it's OK for you to feel that way. We went ahead and made a list of the things we miss the most after having kids. You have our permission to read it in the comfort of your own closet while you munch down on that secret chocolate stash from Halloween last year (it's OK, we all do it).

Read away and know that it's completely normal, natural, and acceptable to feel a sense of loss about these things. It's OK to wish you had some (or all) of these things back. It doesn't make you a monster to feel like you're missing out on something because you *are* missing out. It's part of this crazy motherhood world, and longing for these things again doesn't mean you are a bad mother or that you would trade your kids for anything. We just want you to stand with us in the "we're all human and we have basic needs" arena for a hot second. So, sit back, grab yourself a bite-sized Three Musketeers, and let's really talk this over.

These are things you might miss (and it's totally OK to feel this):

- Sleep, in general.
- Guilt-free and long showers.
- Your pre-baby body (not rock-hard abs, just the pre-baby body that looked and felt fine for an entire week after a simple yoga routine, a 30-minute cycling class, and a couple of salads).
- Spontaneity, in general.
- Having conversations with adults about adult stuff.
- Hot coffee—a whole cup of it all in one glorious sitting.
- Guilt-free glasses of wine. One is fine; one more, not so much! Early bird wake-ups are not a good match for too much of that!
- Being able to cook and clean when you want to, how you want to, if you want to!
- Sneezing, coughing, laughing, and otherwise moving freely, knowing that your bladder is on your team.
- Getting dressed before breakfast, knowing that nobody's mucus, burp, or poop (yes, poop!) will force you to change before leaving the house.
- Leaving your house with only your wallet, phone, and car keys.
- Having an uninterrupted phone conversation at any time of the day.
- Being sick, as in lying in bed and saying, "Oof! I feel terrible! I can barely get out of bed!" and actually staying in bed.
- Silence. Oh, glorious silence.

Motherhood is the ultimate journey. When we become mothers, we move into a wholly different space, and it changes us; it reshapes every element of our being—from the big things to the little ones. The change is huge, it's real, and it forces us to manage our time, efforts, energy, body, emotions, and relationships in entirely new ways. This change is not simple, and it takes much hard work to figure out. For most of us, a lot of trial and error goes into this. There are some things you knew would be affected, and there are other changes or situations you never anticipated encountering, such as this next one.

THE MOST EMBARRASSING CROSSFIT WORKOUT *EVER*, BY Z

My husband is a very hands-on guy, both as a dad and as a partner. During my first pregnancy, after the vomiting died down, we started to get back to our usual workout routine, taking long power walks together every night. After the baby was born, it seemed only natural to get right back to our healthy lifestyle, and a friend had recommended we try out the new CrossFit gym that had just opened up a block away from our apartment. My husband signed us both up. I appreciated his initiative and went along with the plan.

My sister came to stay, and I was glad to get a little time out of the house and do something different; mothering was already starting to get monotonous. We walked over to the gym, met the instructor, and learned what to do and not to do. Then the class started. The very fit and muscular trainer instructed us to take a quick run around the block to start the class. I was laughing with my husband about something, happy I was having this little me time with him.

But as soon as we started running, I felt something start to leak. "Huh! My period here already? Darn, should have worn a Carefree!" I thought. A few more steps, a little more leaking. "Huh! Silly me! I totally thought that you didn't get your period again until after you stopped breastfeeding!"

I slowed down my jog, but something was definitely not right. With every step I took, my panties (and now my tights) kept getting wetter and wetter. I stopped dead in my tracks, feeling a bit of panic. This was way too much blood. My black yoga pants were wet down to the knees. I freaked out and snuck a peek into my tights to see the bloody damage. But there was nothing to be seen. No red. Just pure, crystal clear, transparent liquid. I realized I had completely, absolutely peed on myself at 28 years old. I wanted to die.

A girl ran past me, and I hollered "Hey! Tell my husband that I have to go home for a sec!" and turned around and started walking home. I didn't really know what I was feeling because it was basically too much. I wanted to cry and then crawl under a rock and never see any of these people again. I was embarrassed, frustrated, and just trying to get home as fast as possible to change my clothes.

And that's when I ran into a very hip friend and her cool and good-looking husband. Oh, no. My mind acted quickly. I couldn't stop and say hi because they would smell the pee. But I had to say something; otherwise, I would seem crazy and weird! So, I started to fake jog again, even though I had sworn off any form of running for the rest of my life just two seconds before. I cracked my face into a smile and waved very enthusiastically, "Heeeey guuuuys! Getting some exercise done! To get back to that pre-baby weight! Ha, ha, ha...." and I ran off like a fox scurrying into the woods.

I stormed into my apartment to find my sister there on the couch with my baby. "Hey! How was the cla...."

"I PEED ON MYSELF!" I yelled and went straight into my shower, slamming the door behind me. I was furious. This was not part of the plan. I was OK with the vomiting for three months, the nightly peeing, and the 36 hours of labor. I had put up with the episiotomy and the painful nipples (OK, maybe I complained about the nipples a little bit). But peeing on myself? My life had reached a whole new low!

Moms give up a lot in service to another person. It's completely admirable and astonishing. But birth is just the beginning of what happens through matrescence. The next step is the identity collision.

CHAPTER 3

Identity Collision

For the first few months of motherhood (and sometimes into the early childhood years), many moms are sucked into a cycle of constant caretaking. It's suddenly our responsibility to make sure the baby is eating the right foods, listening to the right songs, and sleeping at the right times. It can feel overwhelming and exhausting.

But some moms have the opposite experience. They don't feel stressed out—or at least they don't show it on the outside. For these moms, everything seems to be under control and without problems.

NOT TO RUB IT IN, BUT...BY M

I coasted through being pregnant and the early years of being a mother without feeling overwhelmed or in over my head, honestly. I kept myself busy with a healthy balance of caring for my kids and running my small business. It never seemed to be hard to squeeze in chores and time with the kids between consulting calls or filming new courses for my online school start-up. I had it all mostly under control, though, because I was lucky.

Through a tight situation of having few options, I had to work with what I had, which was just my computer and a whole lot of wanting to do something with myself. And to make Z hate me a little bit more, I had zero nausea during my pregnancies. I felt great and was able to fully function throughout all four of them.

ME, NOT SO MUCH, BY Z

Motherhood for me could not have been more different than M's kick start. It was constantly pulling me in a hundred directions, and I gave it everything I had. All of my pregnancies were a gory, pukey mess. I tried to keep my head above water, but, somehow, I always felt like I wasn't doing it right. I often told myself that I should have known better, or tried harder, or done something differently. Whenever I stopped by M's house and saw how laid-back everything was and how well-behaved and harmonious M's kids were, I felt completely baffled.

Then, after a few years, the kids got a little older and things started to slow down around my home. I finally felt like I could stop and take a breath. And that's when I found myself starting to wonder, "What happened to me?"

Now I know that I was experiencing an identity collision. That's what happens when your pre-mom identity crashes head-on into your post-mom identity. The sensation of an identity collision is always the same. Mostly, you feel a strange sense of emptiness. It's like something is missing from your life, and you can't quite put a finger on what.

This sensation of emptiness and incompleteness that many moms feel when the craziness starts to die down often means that the woman you were before—the one with a name besides "Mom"—is dying to come out. As you mull over the feeling, trying to figure out what it means and where it came from, you might find that a single question emerges: "Where did I go?" Or, as I put it, "What happened to me?"

Matrescence is a time of reinventing your identity for your role as a mother, just like adolescence was about reinventing your identity for your role as an adult. Existential questions are actually a sign that you're right where you are supposed to be.

Remember, the goal is to move through matrescence successfully, not to get stuck halfway through. That means you need to push forward. Avoiding the hard questions will only slow you down. Sooner or later, they will have to be answered if you want to move forward.

You might realize that little by little, one piece at a time, you've been losing the things that made you, *you*. Each small sacrifice you've made has forced you to give something up.

And now, what's left? That's an identity collision.

Experiencing this sensation doesn't suggest anything negative about you as a person or a mother. And the reason why it happens can be as simple as you have lost yourself in the overpowering love for that new little being so much that your own self-love has taken a back seat.

> *"Every night before bed I tell my daughter, 'I love you so much,' and she always responds 'too much,' and if that doesn't describe motherhood I don't know what does."*
>
> —Tweet by *Holly Loftin* @Bottomofmypurse

Dr. Ashurina Ream, a psychologist who works with moms during pregnancy and postpartum, has an account called @psychedmommy where she helps moms feel more supported.[11] She writes in an Instagram post, "How can overwhelming love and sense of loss coexist?" Then she goes on to write how just because we love our children, it doesn't mean we can't feel a sense of loss. The truth is, according to Dr. Ream, we *have* lost something of our former lives, and it's OK to admit that. But we've gained a lot too. In our experience, some mothers feel like they've lost a part of themselves when they have children, but they're afraid people will judge them if they admit it.

Moms experience this sensation of losing themselves in vastly different ways. Some moms manage to navigate through matrescence without experiencing an identity collision, while other moms do experience it. From our research, we've categorized three main types of mom identities. The first two types usually lead to a violent identity collision on the way through matrescence, but the third type of mom identity can often avoid an identity collision altogether.

MOM IDENTITY #1: OVERACHIEVER MOM

Overachiever Moms plan to do it all. Before getting pregnant, these moms confidently tell themselves they are going to rise through the ranks at their jobs and get the corner office while still picking up the kids from

---

11 "Dr. Ream | Postpartum Support (@Psychedmommy)" Instagram Post, accessed October 7, 2020, https://www.instagram.com/psychedmommy/.

daycare every day on time. They're going to make beautiful babies and then get their pre-pregnancy bodies back—in three months. They're going to have a wildly romantic and intimate relationship with their partner and also be an active member of the PTA.

Their living rooms will look like a spread out of *Better Homes and Gardens*, and their meals will taste as if they were prepared by Martha Stewart herself.

MOM IDENTITY #2: ULTIMATE MOM

Before becoming pregnant, Ultimate Moms look forward to motherhood as the best and most rewarding thing they will ever do. They plan to be the most caring, supportive, and available mothers possible. They will have fun family brunches together on Sundays (with whole grain, sugar-free pancakes, of course). Their brownies will be legendary and loved by all. Their kids will be their masterpieces, their own little Mona Lisas and Sistine Chapels. They will be right there to take care of any and every need. They will kiss every scraped knee, cheer for every soccer goal, cry for every graduation, and say "bless you" for every sneeze.

Of course, these expectations are incredibly unrealistic. Overachiever and Ultimate Moms set particularly high standards for themselves. It's impossible to be perfect at everything, and by expecting that they will be, they are setting themselves up for disappointment.

But the real reason these two mom identities can be problematic is because they both subtly encourage moms to define their worth based on *how good of a mom they are*. They provide two different definitions of what a "good" mom is, but the underlying message is the same: *You're a mom now and being a good one is the most important thing*. This mentality is what sets up Overachiever and Ultimate Moms for a violent identity collision. In many cases, even the Overachiever Moms who manage to achieve everything they said they would and the Ultimate Moms who raise the most amazing children still experience an identity collision. At the root of the problem is a conflict between two identities. Both types of moms have shifted their identity to be fully "mom," staking their happiness on their kids.

We get why this happens. It's *really* hard to look at those kids and not tie your satisfaction to how they are doing. Their wins, losses, struggles, and successes feel like your own. You should definitely be proud of your kids, but staking your happiness on how someone else is doing is not only unfair to the other person, it's also unfair to you. It's a way of surrendering your power to someone else. It also means you've overidentified as a mom, which becomes a problem because no one is *just* a mom. Try to let go of some of your overidentification with your kids (we all have some of it). This brings us to the third type of mom identity.

MOM IDENTITY #3: CASUAL MOM

This type of mom is less identified with her role as a mother and caregiver than the other two mom identities. She sees being a mom as something she *does*, not who she *is*. She thinks of "mom" as part of her identity, but not necessarily the central or most important part. When her kids have problems, she doesn't see them as *her* problems. She can shrug her shoulders and say, "My kid really messed that one up." She maintains her own passions outside of family life and contributes to the world in ways other than only through her kids. She might love every second of being a mom, but she also views herself as much more than only a mom.

THE SILENT TREATMENT

Why do so few moms talk about the identity collision of matrescence? Moms keep silent about the identity collision because we don't want to sound ungrateful or selfish. We don't want to be seen as unfit mothers. Nobody wants a dubious pilot flying the plane, so we continue to move forward, praying that the mountains under us won't scrape our bellies instead of looking at our control panel to see if there are any blinking red lights. It's almost as if we give ourselves the silent treatment and block all emergency exits of communication.

One of the most difficult parts about experiencing an identity collision is that we can each feel like we are the only one going through this. All around us, other moms are so content and happy with their lives. *It must be just me*, we think to ourselves, and then we try to shove down the discomfort and the loss of self that we feel, doubling down on our love of momhood.

"I don't resent being pregnant.... I resent everyone who hasn't been honest. I resent the culture of how much women have to suck it the f--k up and act like everything is fine. I really resent that."

—Amy Schumer[12]

Amy is talking about the fact that she had hyperemesis gravidarum, a condition that affects less than three percent of pregnant women and gives them severe morning sickness.[13] It makes women feel like they have food poisoning for almost their entire pregnancy, and as such, it comes with severe vomiting, nausea, and dizziness. In her documentary series, *Expecting Amy*, she states that she was expected to not talk about it and move forward with her professional demands. She wondered specifically about all of the moms who, unlike her, couldn't afford everything that she could splurge on to feel better and navigate such a hard pregnancy.[14]

This highlights one of the many situations that moms silence during pregnancy and after giving birth, and the parenting books aren't very helpful when it comes to this, either. Pick up any parenting book, and there's a better than good chance it's going to be about the kids—not the parents—as shown by this list of common topics in parenting books:

- How to make my kids stop fighting
- How to raise a secure child
- How to make your baby sleep through the night
- How to have a school-smart, street-smart, marry-the-right-person, or next-Mark-Zuckerberg-smart kid
- How to have a yoga-practicing, chai-green-tea-drinking, peaceful kid

Anybody else exhausted and confused already? Not enough people talk about the inner aspects of being a mom and how easy it is to lose ourselves in all of it. Few people seem to be talking about how becoming a mom can lead to this insane existential crisis of identity when we finally wake up and realize we've been sucked into a mom time warp.

---

12 *Expecting Amy*, directed by Ryan Cunningham and Alexander Hammer, HBO Max, 2020.
13 Traci C. Johnson, "Hyperemesis Gravidarum: Learn About the Causes, Symptoms, and Treatments," WebMD (WebMD, August 30, 2020), https://www.webmd.com/baby/what-is-hyperemesis-gravidarum.
14 *Expecting Amy*, 2020.

"Motherhood, a story of coffee getting cold."
—Unknown mother

HOW LONG IS TEMPORARY AGAIN? BY Z

I had seen my mother be a housewife all of my life, and I was sure I didn't want to be "just a mother" (bear with me that once I did become a mother, I realized that the word "just" in that phrase is completely out of place).

The day my husband and I decided I would stay at home to raise our firstborn, I was 100 percent sure it was temporary. Seven years later, I still hadn't gone back to work on a consistent level. I had always planned to be a working mom, but once my firstborn came with a heart condition and special needs, everything changed. The guilt gobbled me up, spat me out, and left me confused, tired, and lost in my kitchen writing up the grocery list with the last two brain cells available. Life was…um…dull.

Nobody was holding a gun to my head; I could have easily walked into many companies, left my CV, and tried my luck. But the decision to go back to work was not as easy as I had always thought it would be. Would I take an eight-hour-a-day job? Should I get a part-time job? How much money would I be paid for part time? Would it be enough to hire a nanny to take care of the baby while I was away? Plus, with speech therapy, occupational therapy, and physical therapy, I could barely keep up with it all. How would somebody else? But the truth was that I was not happy with myself as a mother and as a woman in that confused state, and I couldn't seem to figure out what was wrong. I was overthinking and beating myself up constantly about what I "should" be doing with my time and how.

For most moms, it is very hard to admit to anyone besides ourselves that it isn't going as well as we had thought it would. We are afraid others will interpret that as, "I don't want to be a mom anymore," which, of course, is *not true*. And it really isn't even about that.

Everyone has moments of longing for the yesterdays of less responsibility. When you're 25, you might think wistfully about your college days when life was so easy. In college, you pine for the times you spent hanging out with your high school friends. In high school, you look with envy at the kindergarteners who get to run around and paint with their fingers all day (for some reason, nobody ever wants to go back to middle school). The point is that it's totally normal to feel regret or longing for a past version of yourself or for easier times—especially in moments when things are particularly hard.

But most of us don't talk about the identity collision; we keep quiet about it. And this is a huge problem, because the message new moms hear most often about motherhood is how great it is, how much they are going to love it, and how fulfilling it will be. This silence about the entire existence of matrescence helps to perpetuate the two unhealthy mom identities, and this sets up more moms for an unexpected identity collision later on.

It's a case of cognitive dissonance, or inconsistent thoughts, beliefs, and attitudes. In simple terms, moms are rationalizing away discontent with their motherhood because they don't think they're supposed to be feeling that way. *Only a bad mom would wish she didn't have kids sometimes. And I'm a good mom. So, I must not feel that way.*

Imagine you go to school for six years in order to get a top job in finance. But then, after three years on the job, it starts to get old. It's not so exciting anymore, and you're bored. When people ask how your job is going, though, you say, "It's great! I love it." The fact that you spent six years studying to be an accountant is incompatible with the fact that you don't enjoy the work. So, you convince yourself that you actually do like the work. *Hey, it's really great pay, the hours aren't bad, the benefits are nice, and some of it is kind of rewarding.*

It's impossible to change the fact that you've already spent six years preparing yourself for this job. So, your brain focuses on trying to convince yourself that you actually *do* like the job. Eventually, however, there's going to be a collision.

As we become moms, our cognitive dissonance leads to some consistent patterns. We convince ourselves that we can't or shouldn't want anything more or different because of thoughts like these:

- I tried so long to get pregnant; I really can't complain.
- It's selfish to want anything different.
- We already put so much time and energy into this.
- I love being with my kids, and when I don't, it's because I'm doing it wrong.

- Staying at home really is a luxury.
- Having a job and having kids really is a luxury.
- It took so long to adopt that my friends or family will think I'm crazy or a bad person.
- We're not grateful enough.
- How could we possibly not feel anything but pure, sheer happiness and love 100 percent of the time?

EVERYTHING IS FINE! BY M

A week after having my first daughter, I received an email from a friend who had had twins a couple of months before. She was several years older than I was, and since I had become a mom a bit before most of my friends had, I didn't have many friends my age with babies. So, it was nice to receive a message from someone who was already surfing the stage, and I was happy to know we would be in touch. In her email, she was as joyful as always. She asked me if I was feeling great, living with the immense happiness from having my baby, and loving motherhood.

As I read her words, an overwhelming feeling of inadequacy started to seep in. "Crap," I thought, "Why am I not so joyful and exploding with the happiness she says I should feel?" The truth was that I was incredibly happy, but I was also feeling deeply exhausted from skipped sleep, a bit claustrophobic with this new deal of breastfeeding and losing my physical independence to a little baby, and simply silent inside, observing myself and trying to master this whole baby world I was so new to.

How was I going to answer back that this change was harder than I had expected? She had twins, and she had given birth in a faraway country! I was still in Chile at the time, and she had already been relocated to Washington, D.C. Yet, somehow, she found this experience to be wonderful and amazing. How could I be so ungrateful and petty? I sheepishly answered back, "Yes! Everything is just fine!" All I could manage to write about the actual truth was, "I'm writing this email between feedings," and left it at that.

It was years later that I realized that this silent treatment was precisely what had prevented me from truly telling her how I felt. I was not able to really talk about how I felt, and instead I wrote a clichéd email with the word "fine," hoping that that was what everyone expected me to say.

By not being able to fully admit our internal struggles to ourselves, we've also made any public discussion of matrescence practically taboo. We need to be able to start talking about the experience of becoming a mother. As moms, we need to talk about our *whole selves*, not just our mom side.

This is a really complex issue that didn't start with us. It's a problem that's been around for a considerably long time. At the root of the identity collision is a reliance on unreal cultural standards for motherhood. But where did these standards come from?

CHAPTER 4

Mom Shaming

If expectations about motherhood are at the root of the matrescence identity collision, then it makes sense to ask where these expectations come from in the first place. How did we develop the Overachiever and Ultimate Mom prototypes? Why do so many of us start to unconsciously define ourselves based on our role as a mother? To answer these questions, we have to take a trip back in history for a second.

It was in the early 1900s that the word *parenting* was first used as a verb.[15] We then started seeing the true evolution of the modern family and the parental roles we think of today as mom and dad.[16] The idea that moms are soft, loving, and run the home while dads are tough, demanding, and don't talk much was largely continued during this time.

As the 1920s rolled around, child labor laws began to be passed,[17] and mandatory childhood education was becoming more widely enforced.[18] Also, Sigmund Freud's new field of psychology was starting to gain popularity and with it came the idea that parents play a critical role in child

---

15 "Parenting," Merriam-Webster, accessed October 9, 2020, https://www.merriam-webster.com/dictionary/parenting.
16 Caroline Mills Hinkle, "Creating Dad: The Remaking of Middle-Class Fatherhood in the United States," PhD diss. (University of California, Berkeley, 2011).
17 "The Child Labor Amendment, 1924–1934," CQ Researcher, accessed October 12, 2020, http://library.cqpress.com/cqresearcher/document.php?id=cqresrre1934030300.
18 Michael S. Katz, *A History of Compulsory Education* (Bloomington, IN: Phi Delta Kappa, 1976): 21.

development.[19] By the 1930s, women were entering the workforce and getting college educations in higher numbers.[20, 21] As a result, the number of children per household started to drop.[22]

From the 1940s through the 1960s, the middle class boomed along with the suburbs.[23] The US post-WWII was rolling in dough,[24] and by the 1950s, a single salary could often support an entire household.[25] Men came back from the war and reclaimed many jobs that women had taken over, leading to a backslide in rights for women.[26]

And that's when gender roles grew more rigid.[27] Suddenly pink was for girls, and blue was for boys.[28] Parents now needed to buy different toys, clothes, and bedding for boys and girls. Parental responsibilities started to become more strictly defined, and this led to a solidification of the breadwinner family model, with men paying the bills and women taking care of the home.[29]

A couple of decades later, women were finally able to have both a career

---

19 Geoffrey H. Steer," Freudianism and Child-Rearing in the Twenties," *American Quarterly* 20, no. 4 (1968): 759–767, https://doi.org/10.2307/2711406.
20 Elisabeth Jacob and Kate Bahn, "Women's History Month: U.S. women's labor force participation," Washington Center for Equitable Growth," March 22, 2019, https://equitablegrowth.org/womens-history-month-u-s-womens-labor-force-participation/.
21 Margaret A. Nash and Lisa Romero, "'Citizenship for the College Girl': Challenges and Opportunities in Higher Education for Women in the United States in the 1930s," *Teachers College Record* 114 (2012).
22 Mark Mather, "The Decline in U.S. Fertility," Populations Reference Bureau (PRB), July 18, 2012, https://www.prb.org/us-fertility/.
23 Claire Suddath, "A Brief History of The Middle Class," *TIME*, February 27, 2009, http://content.time.com/time/nation/article/0,8599,1882147,00.html.
24 Jordan Weissmann, "60 Years of American Economic History, Told in 1 Graph," *The Atlantic*, August 23, 2012, https://www.theatlantic.com/business/archive/2012/08/60-years-of-american-economic-history-told-in-1-graph/261503/.
25 "Income of Families and Persons in the United States: 1950," United States Census Bureau, March 25, 1952, https://www.census.gov/library/publications/1952/demo/p60-009.html#:~:text=Average%20family%20income%20in%201950,the%20Census%2C%20Department%20of%20Commerce.
26 "Women and Work After World War II," PBS, accessed October 12, 2020, https://www.pbs.org/wgbh/americanexperience/features/tupperware-work/.
27 "Women and Work After World War II."
28 Susan Stamberg, "Girls Are Taught To 'Think Pink,' But That Wasn't Always So," NPR, April 1, 2014, https://www.npr.org/2014/04/01/297159948/girls-are-taught-to-think-pink-but-that-wasnt-always-so.
29 "Mrs. America: Women's Roles in the 1950s," PBS, accessed October 12, 2020, https://www.pbs.org/wgbh/americanexperience/features/pill-mrs-america-womens-roles-1950s/.

and children if they wanted, but usually the career had to be squeezed in before or after tending to the kids.[30] The parenting industry erupted during the 1970s and parenting books appeared everywhere.[31] Family life started to become a bit more fluid, but for the most part, moms still did the majority of caregiving and nurturing, not to mention cooking and housework.[32] The feminist movement of the 1970s was revived in the 1990s with a vengeance.[33] Technological advances like cell phones and the Internet started to evolve at a faster pace, and soon women had more access to each other's lives.[34] By the 2010s, technology and social media were exploding,[35] and all of a sudden, we had a thousand more moms to compare ourselves with and see all the ways we were constantly falling short.

Researchers Margaret Quinlan and Bethany Johnson wrote a book on mom shaming called *You're doing it wrong! Mothering, Media and Medical Expertise* and talk about how the information overload and the number of experts in every field, from lactation consultants, pediatricians, moms of various children, or older children than the ones you have, can sometimes turn off our inner motherly instinct. It can even trail us away from paying attention to what we're actually doing at that very moment. Our kids need us to pay attention to what's going on now.

There's also a stream of information that is being commercialized, which is even more dangerous, because there are people behind the information trying to profit from our attention as moms. So whatever they're talking about or selling, trust us when we say they'll try to convince you that the product they represent will be the new staple of being a "good," "healthy,"

---

30 Lesley Lazin Novack and David R. Novack, "Being female in the eighties and nineties: Conflicts between new opportunities and traditional expectations among white, middle-class, heterosexual college women," *Sex Roles* 35 (1996), https://doi.org/10.1007/BF01548175.
31 Claire Cain Miller, "The Relentlessness of Modern Parenting," *New York Times*, December 25, 2018, https://www.nytimes.com/2018/12/25/upshot/the-relentlessness-of-modern-parenting.html.
32 Jonathan Gershuny and John P. Robinson, "Historical Changes in the Household Division of Labor," *Demography* 25, no. 4 (November 1988): 537–552, https://doi.org/10.2307/2061320.
33 "The Third Wave of Feminism," *Encyclopedia Britannica*, accessed October 12, 2020, https://www.britannica.com/topic/feminism/The-third-wave-of-feminism.
34 Tiffanie Darke, "The 1990s: When Technology Upended Our World," History, updated January 31, 2019, https://www.history.com/news/90s-technology-changed-culture-internet-cellphones.
35 Esteban Ortiz-Ospina, "The rise of social media," Our World in Data, September 18, 2019, https://ourworldindata.org/rise-of-social-media.

"educated," "original," or whatever adjective you're looking for to feel satisfied in this new field of parenting. They'll talk about the problem that this product fixes as a much bigger issue than it usually is, just for the sake of the sale. "This is the safest crib available on the market today." The words "nontoxic" applied to every single toy produces internal alarms in all of us. Then comes the stock photos of the Pinterest mom working from home with a toddler on her lap that some ad for a bank or continuing education program might sell. "We get your reality; we're here for you." But the message that the ad is giving off can produce a false idea that it's actually super simple to cram for an online MBA with a toddler on your lap. Trust us when we say, this book was written in the wee hours of the morning—before 7am, when no toddler could sit on our laps—or late at night when everyone was sound asleep. Not saying someone couldn't pull a book off with bouncing babies on the knee, but we do consider the latter a bit less stressful and more productive.

The pressure can be very overwhelming. Many reasons can show us how we got here, but the important thing is to know what your "here" is and what you want to do. Your role as a mom doesn't have to be the most important thing about you unless you choose it to be so. Studies show that we are most fulfilled when we have multiple roles to shift between every day.[36] Being a mom can be just one basket to put your eggs in—a great one—but one out of many possibilities, and it doesn't have to be the only thing you get excited about. In fact, it shouldn't be, so let's go build us a couple more baskets.

GUILTY AS CHARGED

> *"Don't ever judge a mum for looking at her phone while her kids play. She's probably Googling private schools or raw dessert recipes. Just kidding. She's scrolling Instagram and deserves three minutes of peace."*
>
> —*Unknown*

Moms today are better educated than any other generation in history, and we have more information at our fingertips than ever before. You can

---

[36] "Modern family roles improve life satisfaction for parents," Science Daily, October 9, 2019, https://www.sciencedaily.com/releases/2019/10/191008104647.htm.

find many moms who get into heated discussions on social media about the "right" and "wrong" way to raise a child. There's always a mom who will post a comment such as, "I breastfed my child until he was X months/years old because I wanted to be sure that he had all of the nutrients to have a fully developed brain."

These comments written and read in the most innocent way can sometimes put us in a situation of comparison whether we want to or not. So those of us who dared give our kids an ounce of something other than "liquid gold" have somehow stunted their brain development? Only breastfed kids will get into Ivy League schools? And here we were stressing out about getting them to learn their ABCs and 123s! Why even bother?!

Mom shaming has always been around. It's hard enough being a little bit sleep-deprived and patience-deprived at all times without our ever-so-eloquent mother-in-law offering some unsolicited parenting advice: "You know, I think you should really try to have [your six-year-old daughter] clean her room before she comes down to dinner." Even worse are the indirect questions: "They sure get sick a lot, don't they? Do you think it's a good idea to keep sending them to daycare?"

And then along comes social media, all fun and ready to connect us and let us be more together, and boom, we have an eagle eye into the life of the perfect, daily-fresh-batch-of-cookies-baking mom with the perfect hair and clean kids. It's hard not to wonder how she does it. We maybe even entertain the thought of getting some of the stuff she has in her house, perhaps try out all of those activities with our own kids, and eventually fall into the trap of comparing apples with oranges.

For example, when Chrissy Teigen posted a video of her son Miles's first steps on Instagram, some commenters felt the need to shame Chrissy, criticizing the toddler's proximity to the edge of a marble bathtub.[37] Do you really need strangers to come along and point out what a terrible mom you are? We don't.

Mom shame can be more subtle, too. Consider a comment like "I only buy my baby organic milk from Whole Foods." People may be saying these things in a very innocent way, to simply share a fact about their lives, but we still feel mom shame.

---

37 Chrissy Teigen, Instagram post, @chrissyteigen, July 30, 2019, https://www.instagram.com/p/B0j6jHbnvq8/?utm_source=ig_embed.

Sometimes, mom shaming comes from a mom who is actually shaming herself, so we have to listen and have our antenna up and working to catch those words the other mom may speak out of her own fear. If we don't, then we might absorb these comments as something we "should" be doing, and the consequences could be devastating. We might end up in the "I'm a bad mom" arena, and that serves no one.

Sometimes we even do our own internal mom shaming. Maybe we read a book about how to manage our child's emotions, and we start to beat ourselves up for not using some of these strategies sooner. Or maybe we try a new summer camp with our kid, and it backfires. Then we rethink every step that got us there and what we did wrong instead of being our own best friend and reminding ourselves that we've got a lot going on, we're doing our best, and that this step back has gotten us two steps forward in the mom world.

> *"We had our second child, our daughter, in 2004. I further embraced motherhood, adding modifiers to claim it as my new identity: I'm a home-schooling mama of two, a SAHM (stay-at-home mom), and a part-time freelancer. I'm a breast-feeding mom. A home-birth mom. A Buddhist mom. I'm a vegetarian natural mama who rejects fast food, plastic toys, screen time, and mainstream everything. There were times when I hugged my new adjectives tighter than my babies—maybe because I couldn't hold on to who I used to be. Everything was slippery."*
>
> —Leslie J. Davis[38]

WELCOME TO THE WORLD OF MOM GUILT

First, we'll discuss the difference between guilt and shame. As Brené Brown explains in her excellent TED Talk: "Shame is a focus on self, guilt is a focus on behavior. Shame is, 'I am bad.' Guilt is, 'I did something bad.' How many of you, if you did something that was hurtful to me, would be willing to say, 'I'm sorry. I made a mistake?' How many of you would be willing to say that? Guilt: 'I'm sorry. I made a mistake.' Shame: 'I'm sorry.

---

[38] Leslie J. Davis, "Motherhood gave me an identity crisis. Solving it was simple, but it wasn't easy," The *Washington Post*, October 4, 2018, https://www.washingtonpost.com/news/parenting/wp/2018/10/04/motherhood-gave-me-an-identity-crisis-solving-it-was-simple-but-it-wasnt-easy/.

I am a mistake.'"[39]

Brené continues to say that shame is directly connected to addiction, depression, violence, aggression, bullying, suicide, and eating disorders. "Here's what you even need to know more: Guilt is inversely correlated with those things. The ability to hold something we've done, or failed to do, up against who we want to be is incredibly adaptive. It's uncomfortable, but it's adaptive."[40]

Mom guilt is a special kind of guilt, and it's completely toxic. Mom guilt is about feeling bad that you didn't do something for your kids as well as you were "supposed" to—in other words, as well as you expected yourself to do it. It is wondering whether you just messed up your child for life by feeding him the wrong food or not signing her up for the right after-school program or working late instead of rushing straight home to play. Mom guilt doesn't come from inside of you, like normal guilt. Instead, it's imposed on you from the outside—and then you internalize it and take it on. That's how it can turn into shame and take you even deeper down the rabbit hole of identity loss.

Mom guilt is based on other people's expectations, but we beat ourselves up when we fail to meet those expectations. Mom guilt can really pull you into a tailspin fast. We're here to tell you that this type of guilt, while completely normal to feel, is not helpful to wallow in. In fact, it may sometimes turn into one of the most difficult emotions for us to manage.

In recent decades, as women have become more liberated, our society has continued to add more and more new expectations onto moms without taking away any of the old ones. We're being overloaded with external pressures and shoulds, and it leads to a massive amount of guilt when we can't live up to it all.

THE POISONED STRAWBERRY, BY Z

I experience this mom guilt every day in one form or another. In fact, I recently managed to feel guilty when I couldn't find organic strawberries at the grocery store. I stopped dead in my tracks when I got to the strawberry display and there were no organic strawberries left. Those healthy, green organic labels

---

[39] Brené Brown, "Listening to shame," TED, recorded March 2012, https://www.ted.com/talks/brene_brown_listening_to_shame#t-14298.
[40] Ibid.

were nowhere to be found, but I needed those organic strawberries. Every morning my husband makes the kids a banana, orange juice, pear, and strawberry smoothie. We run a tight ship when it comes to routines and meal plans. The days we run out of strawberries, the kids sometimes pass on the healthy drink to start off their day, and it's one thing my husband and I like to count on for the kids to get in their fruits for the day.

Organic versus nonorganic had never been an issue for me. I had heard that in the US it's best to go organic with certain products in the meat or dairy department, but I had never heard about the dangers in the fruit and veggie aisle. And when I saw the prices, I decided to wing it with the nonorganic. I didn't have the budget.

Then one day during a casual conversation next to the soccer field, some moms were commenting on which nonorganic fruits and veggies were safe to buy. At one point, Regina, one of the moms who knew a bit more on the subject, said something about strawberries. I asked her what she was talking about. "When it comes to strawberries," she explained, "you absolutely have to go organic. If there isn't an organic version to buy, you're better off never buying strawberries again. It's literally poisoned with pesticides and it can't be washed off before eating." I wanted to buy organic, but I had to confess that I had sometimes done the latter.

So, when I stood there staring at the regular, conventional, nonorganic strawberries, my mom guilt flared up massively. I realized that something inside me was getting tense and agitated. Buying the nonorganic ones was basically a crime against my children, right? I knew how bad they were for my kids now. I knew, because Regina had said so. I couldn't go back to blissfully "poisoning" my children! But then I thought about the kids whining for an entire week every morning. My kids barely eat food from a box or a can, so couldn't I let this slide just for once?

I took a deep breath and picked up a box of strawberries without even looking. I couldn't bear it. I placed them into my shopping cart and, for a tiny second, felt I was placing a hand grenade in there, literally. Then, I wheeled myself out of the produce aisle and went to find the rest of the items on my list. But the feelings of guilt kept gnawing at me for days.

Mom guilt is real, and it is diverse. It can be as simple as feeling bad about picking up a pizza for your kids on the way home because you're too tired to cook, or as complicated as deciding whether or not to go part-time after your maternity leave is up. It creeps into everything if you don't call it by its name.

> *"Guilt management can be just as important as time management for mothers."*
> —Sheryl Sandberg, CEO of Facebook[41]

The most difficult thing is that mom guilt feels just like regular healthy guilt. It uses the same brain circuits, and it can be difficult to tell the two apart. But there is one way you can start to get a bit more control over these feelings—and it starts with debunking your mom expectations.

IT'S SUCH A SHAME

We've seen that mom shame is toxic and that it stems from expectations about motherhood that have been slowly layered on to women since the Victorian era. The expectations that seem to cause the most guilt for moms today include the following:

1. Moms should be kind, caring, and loving, never pushy or forceful.
2. Moms should know everything there is to know about parenting.
3. Moms should always put the needs of the family first, even above themselves.

THERE'S ALWAYS ONE PARENT, BY M

A few weeks ago, I was rushing to get my son to school on time. It was one of those days where everything seemed to be running behind schedule. He woke up late, it took forever to get out the door, and traffic was crawling along the freeway. I had less than an hour to drop him off at school and get home in time to run a live webinar with 25 new students in my online marketing school.

When I finally pulled up to the front door, school had already begun and there were no teachers in sight at the morning drop-off. "Rats," I thought, then quickly parked in the already empty parking lot (except for the teachers' vehi-

---

[41] Sheryl Sandberg, *Lean In: Women, Work, and the Will to Lead* (New York: Alfred A. Knopf, 2013): 168.

cles) and rolled him out of my car. Time was of the essence. I looked at the clock and realized I absolutely couldn't afford to spend more than five minutes inside.

Walking into the school, I pulled my son along by the wrist, urging him forward. The thwap-thwap of my sandals echoed through the deserted hallway. There was not a single student or teacher lingering at the lockers. Strange.

As we rounded the corner and walked past the administrative offices, I marveled at how quiet the whole school was. It was only five minutes past 8:30 a.m.! It seemed like a bit of a miracle that all the kids had settled in and gotten to work so quickly. *This school certainly is efficient*, I thought to myself.

That's when the principal, Ms. Anne, stepped into the hallway and frowned as she saw my son and me walking along.

"Hello, Ms. Anne," I said, wondering if maybe I could just drop the kid off with her and run, "we're a bit late, so I'm trying to get him to class. Can you help?"

"I'm sorry," Ms. Anne said, "but there is no school today. It is a Wednesday, but today is teacher planning day. We sent out an email last week."

"Oh, my gosh, I totally forgot!" I said, quickly adjusting my mental timeline leading up to the webinar.

"Don't worry!" Principal Anne effused with elementary school warmth. "You shouldn't feel bad about this. There is always a parent who doesn't get the memo. You're not the first, and I'm sure you won't be the last."

"Well, I'm glad you were here to at least let me know what's going on!" I half-joked, preparing our exit. "Have a great day."

I hustled back to the car with my son, where I burst out laughing at myself and took a few deep breaths to calm down before heading home for the webinar. I had just enough time left to set him up in the playroom before updating the slides.

I smiled, remembering Anne's words, "You shouldn't feel bad about this." Actually, I hadn't even thought to worry or feel bad. I just had too much going on, and this wasn't a big deal. This was a time in my life where my chips were spread all over the place, and this screwup wasn't a blow to my ego; it was simply a funny story to tell at dinnertime.

THE DARK SIDE TO HELPING MOTHERS OUT

We started to wonder how often other moms experienced incidents of mom shame. Are moms hit with these types of situations constantly? How do moms cope with this? How can we help moms be ready for this, and how can we keep the kids away from these confrontations that may produce feelings of sorrow and insecurity?

> *"No one can make you feel inferior without your consent."*
> —Attributed to *Eleanor Roosevelt*

In today's world, women have broken through a lot of the expectations that used to hold us back. But for some reason, that hasn't happened for moms. Today, a woman can be sexy, caring, domineering, nice, a badass, or your fun BFF. She can dress and act however she wants, work in any industry she wants, and be as outspoken or quiet as she wants. The possibilities are nearly endless—for *women*.

But can moms be sexy? *Ew, weird. Nope, not part of the mom role.* Can they be messy? *Well, that's not very smart; they'd lose all of the pacifiers every day.* Domineering? *Hmm, that doesn't sound very mom-like either, unless she's defending her kid and then it's OK.* It's almost as if the second a woman becomes a mom, society rolls back most of the options for what she can and can't be, or at least society thinks they can have an opinion over her. We plop her right back in the middle of those Victorian-era expectations. This is why there are still a lot of feelings around mom staying home with the kids versus going back to work full time. Society—and even many women—have a hard time remembering moms are women, too.

> *"It felt like the TV and the movies I was watching about motherhood represented it in this real one-dimensional light. It was either this broad comedy or it was this sort of after-school special type of thing. I wasn't seeing a lot of three-dimensional, fleshed out moms who were still sexy and smart and interesting."*
> —Catherine Reitman, actress, writer, and producer of *Workin' Moms*[42]

---

[42] "Catherine Reitman Is the Consummate Workin' Mom," *Mom Brain* podcast, episode 32, May 20, 2020.

As moms, we are expected to put other people before ourselves. But thinking of others before ourselves is not the key to happiness. In fact, it can be the end of us. That's why they always tell us on airplanes to put our own mask on first before helping others. If they didn't tell us that, adults might struggle with the kids' masks and lose consciousness. Then we wouldn't be able to put on our own masks.

As soon as we become pregnant, we shift from being a woman to being a mom. Matrescence begins, and our identity enters a state of flux as we experiment with what type of mom identity we want to have. For the first few months after birth, we get completely overwhelmed, and it's really hard to even catch our breath and realize what's happening to us. But once we can come up for air, we realize our Rubik's Cube has shifted.

We're now part of a coveted club, and other members will take it upon themselves to police us and make sure we're doing a good job. As moms, we can get shamed at any time and from any direction without warning. Usually it comes from other moms. One minute we're minding our own business and the next we're being told that we're a terrible mother by a complete stranger. It happens on social media, at the grocery store, at the zoo, and anywhere else we might be seen with our family.

If you aren't feeling guilty about something already, don't worry, just go out in public and another mom will be happy to come along and point out what you're doing wrong.

PUT THE CHIPS DOWN, MA'AM, AND PLACE YOUR HANDS WHERE I CAN SEE THEM, BY M

A few months ago, I took my family to the beach. It was turning out to be a perfect spring day. The kids were out of school on one of those unpredictable school holidays and everyone in my house felt like going to the beach. The kids all changed into their swimsuits while I packed up the sunscreen, towels, sun umbrellas, pails, and shovels into the minivan, and then we took off for the beach.

I just forgot one thing: snacks! Not more than an hour after arriving at the beach, my second child asked for something to eat. Then, moments later, I got a second snack request. Then a third.

"Do you guys want to go home and make some food?" I asked the kids, "Or

just eat something quick from the snack stand and stay here for a while?"

The answer was unanimous: Stay! I marched the kids over to the only concession stand to pick up some water and snacks. Predictably, the only snacks available came in shiny, brightly colored foil bags stamped with logos like Cheetos, Doritos, and Lay's. There was no fresh fruit anywhere in sight. I decided it was worth it to get some unhealthy snacks, just this once, so the kids could keep playing on the beach. I bought some chips and passed them around.

The kids squealed with glee and happily munched away, their fingertips turning bright orange. I smiled and opened a bag for myself. I was happy with myself, the situation under control. One mom point for me. The kids were being goofy and having a great time. It was a perfect day.

"Excuse me?"

I looked up to see a slightly older woman approaching with a scowl on her face. "Honey, I just have to tell you those are terrible for the kids," the woman said. "Do you know what kind of nutritional value is in those?"

Blindsided by this stranger, I could only respond, "Ummm...."

And before I could say anything else, the woman continued, "None! They are pure crap. You shouldn't let your kids have those."

Not in the mood to explain my entire nutritional philosophy to the woman or get into an argument, I smiled, said "OK," and quickly pivoted away from the woman to head back to the beach.

Thankfully, after I calmed down from the weird incident, I was able to see this for what it was: mom shaming.

Mom guilt isn't the only thing that keeps you trapped and pressures you to conform to mom expectations; there's also mom shaming. You can usually rely on another mom, dad, or complete stranger to come along and point out exactly what you're doing wrong. It's like a never-ending SAT exam that we all put each other through for some weird reason. Apparently, high school is never really over.

Why do we feel the need to shame each other? Why is it that even when we've let go of mom expectations for ourselves, we still continue to hold other moms accountable to those expectations? After all, if there's anyone who knows how bad a day can get as a mom, it's other moms!

Mom blogger Karen Johnson sat in front of her computer one day and went on a famous "rant" that was shared and commented over 30,000 times on the Internet. She wrote on what makes a good mom, the one that gave birth in the hospital or the one in the bathtub. The one who only buys organic or the one who feeds her kids junk food every once in a while. The one who drinks wine sometimes even in front of their kids or the one that doesn't drink anything at all. Johnson states that all of these are "good moms," and she continues to say how we have to start celebrating ourselves as "good moms" no matter how you do it or who you are. She writes "Parenthood is so incredibly hard, we are often full of self-doubt already, and then we have to face criticisms from others. How great would it be if we all gave each other some grace and support instead? And realize that there are so many types of 'good moms?'"[43]

THAT'S GOOD ENOUGH!

Nobody is perfect. We want all moms to be perfect, yet perfect is a title that varies a lot in every family. Love yourself for who you are, love your past self for who you were, and love your future self for who you will turn out to be.

Someone will always have something to say. Let this not be you, and let it not crumble you down. There's enough external and internal pressure in being a mother without adding to it.

To sum it all up, we want to share a quote from Dr. Donald Winnicott, a pediatrician and psychoanalyst in mid-twentieth century Britain:

"A mother is neither good nor bad nor the product of illusion, but is a separate and independent entity: The good-enough mother… starts off with an almost complete adaptation to her infant's needs, and as time proceeds, she adapts less and less completely, gradually, according to the infant's growing ability to deal with her failure. Her failure to adapt to every need of the child helps them adapt to external realities."[44]

---

[43] Melissa Willets, "Mom's Post Calling for the End of Mom Shaming Is Taking Over the Internet," Parents.com, July 21, 2017, https://www.parents.com/toddlers-preschoolers/everything-kids/moms-post-calling-for-the-end-of-mom-shaming-is-taking-over/.

[44] D. W. Winnicott, "Transitional objects and transitional phenomena; a study of the first not-me possession," *International Journal of Psychoanalysis* 34 (1953): 89–97.

This concept of a good-enough mother comes from Winnicott's observations of thousands of babies and their mothers, which helped him to discover that children benefit from mothers who frustrate them in manageable ways. Children need their mothers or primary caretakers to fail them in tolerable ways on a regular basis so they can learn to live in an imperfect world. Even if you could be perfect, therefore, it wouldn't be good for your kids.

So, relax, grab your cup of coffee, and just be the best mom you can be, because mom guilt and mom shaming are not going anywhere. Let go of those unrealistic standards and expectations. You've got this.

CHAPTER 5

Going All-In

"Becoming a mother is like discovering the existence of a strange new room in the house where you already live."

—*Sarah Walker,* artist

In the world of high-stakes poker tournaments, going all-in means staking your entire stack of chips on a single hand. It means the payouts can be massive and game changing, but if you lose, you'll be wiped out. Poker players can't afford to lose when they are all-in. That's why they won't go all-in on a hand unless they are certain they can win. The moment a player says "I'm all-in" is very intense, and you can feel the tension in the room as the dealer flips over the next card. The emotions of everyone at the table run very high.

What we've realized about matrescence is that the pressures levelled at women during this time cause many moms to go all-in on motherhood. They play all of their identity chips on being a mom instead of spreading their bets around. This is risky because it can cause motherhood to start taking over your life. Like the quote from Sarah Walker, it's great that you found that new room in your house, but don't forget to keep the door unlocked to catch some air from time to time. If you go all-in as a mom, you'll be *extremely* excited and satisfied when your child gets an A or is picked for the big team. You'll feel on top of the world during your "great mom" moments, like when you remember to bring a snack or intuitively sense that your child needs to talk about something important. You went all-in on being a mom and won. Boo-yah!

However, the opposite can just as easily occur. Going all-in on motherhood also means your kids' losses, setbacks, and failures will hit you especially hard. When your child has a terrible day, gets in trouble at school, fails a test, or loses the big game, it can hurt you deeply. There's also the social aspect of winning that we all want our kids to enjoy. Who doesn't want their kid to have good friends and to have fun? But when your kid doesn't get invited to a friend's house or maybe doesn't feel comfortable leaving your side when the rest of the kids do, it can get complicated for us, and our emotional management challenge is to help them come out on the other side feeling stronger and having learned something. And finally, if someone makes a scornful comment about the way you are raising your child, it can simply feel like a complete slap in the face.

Sometimes we even try to "repair" our own past by living through our children's life challenges. In this case, it's not the kid who's insecure; it's us. It's not the teenager who's traumatized; it's us. Projecting our own troubles onto our kids can be a horrible recipe for disaster. These actions and feelings tend to be the ones that push us to have helicopter or overprotective mom tendencies. It blinds us to the natural process that a developing social life requires. We remember how we used to have a great group of friends as kids, and we expect our kids to develop the same peer group overnight. We forget the trips and falls we suffered and only see the goal. So when our own child has a bad semester or a bad year, we can spiral into a panic that our child will be left socially excluded and start to interfere in an unhealthy or unproductive sort of way.

In the game of poker, you sometimes have no choice but to go all-in. Similarly, during the early days of motherhood, it's nearly impossible to keep your post-pregnancy and baby from taking over your life. That can work for a short time, but eventually you'll want to find balance. Putting all of your identity chips in any one category is risky. Keep reading and we'll give you a few tips on how this redistribution of chips can be pulled off in a stress-free yet conscious way to ensure an actual impact in your life.

What is this word *identity* all about? Psychologist Dr. Bruce A. Bracken suggested in 1995 that there are six specific areas that create your identity:

- Social: the ability to interact with others
- Competence: the ability to meet basic needs
- Affect: the awareness of emotional states

- Physical: feelings about looks, health, physical condition, and overall appearance
- Academic: success or failure in school
- Family: how well one functions within the family unit[45]

From a young age, humans are involved in multiple social circles and activities. As a young child, you might have your family social circle, your neighborhood social circle, and preschool or elementary school social circle. Then, as you mature into an adolescent, you start to spread your identity chips around between family, neighbors, sports, classes, clubs, work, and volunteering. If you're not having a good time on the soccer team, it's OK because you have an interest in chemistry, great friends, and a really fun job at the local ice cream shop. You can afford to make a few bad bets when your chips are spread out.

As you get older, however, the number of places you have available to distribute your identity chips grows smaller. You have to choose between what to focus on and what to let go. This is a completely normal part of growing up; you can't do everything in life. The process of becoming an adult is largely about discovering the most rewarding roles for yourself.

IT DOESN'T JUST HAPPEN TO MOMS

Lewis Howes was a football player who had an identity collision after going all-in on his athletic career. Growing up in poverty, Howes didn't have many positive things going on in his life. He was depressed, had trouble in school, was lonely, and assumed he would one day end up in jail like his brother who was busted for selling drugs. Football was the one area where Howes excelled. He loved the sport and was naturally gifted.

For college, Howes chose a school where he could play football. After graduation, he decided to play on an arena league team, where he earned $250 per week. He was gradually betting all of his chips on football. When Howes broke his wrist in 2007, he was immediately cut from his team and had no money. All of a sudden, he could no longer play the game that had been his entire life. Howes was jobless and without skills or work experience, and the economy was headed into a major recession.

---

45 Bruce A. Bracken, *Handbook of Self-Concept: Developmental, Social, and Clinical Considerations* (New York: John Wiley & Sons, 1995).

Thankfully, and with a little bit of outside-the-box thinking, Howes was eventually able to learn some skills and start his own business. He now has a huge following with his *School of Greatness* podcast and community. It took him awhile to regroup, rethink, and re-create his identity from scratch after his injury. Howes is a great victory story in this era because without having to go back to college or go to a 9-to-5 job, he was able to turn his life around, recover all of those chips that he had put in football, and start shuffling them around.

> *"Great parenting—that creates truly happy kids—is more about letting go than holding on too tightly."*
> —*Megan Meeker*, MD, pediatrician, author, speaker, @megmeekermd[46]

Going all-in on an identity is easy to do. When something is working for you, it's natural to lean into it. And as long as your bet is paying off, you look like a huge success to the outside world. But it's fragile. Sooner or later, you'll lose a hand and be wiped out, just like Lewis Howes.

When you adopt an all-in attitude toward motherhood, there is a tendency to measure your success and self-worth by looking at how well your kids are doing—just as an athlete might measure his or her self-worth based on recent athletic performance. When you're winning, you feel great. Unfortunately, however, life is in a constant state of flux, and kids are certainly no exception. They will experience major ups and downs as they discover the world and become their own people. As they get older, kids will adopt their own ideas about what a good life looks like—and their ideas might be radically different from yours.

One of the biggest problems with betting all of your chips on your mom role is the risk of overidentification. As you begin to stake more of your self-worth on your ability to be a great mom, your children's successes become vital to your self-esteem. You might start to overidentify with your kids. This leads to one of the most talked-about parenting phenomena of the last decade: helicopter parenting.

---

[46] Meg Meeker, "Are You a Great Parent, or Are You Overparenting?" *Meeker Parenting Blog*, December 17, 2016, https://www.meekerparenting.com/blog/great-parent-overparenting.

THE PSYCHOLOGY BEHIND HELICOPTER AND SNOWPLOW PARENTING

Recently, helicopter parenting and snowplow parenting have become buzzwords that are (in our opinion) thrown around way too much by media pundits and parenting experts the world over. A helicopter parent hovers just overhead and interferes with tasks in their child's lives that they are already capable of doing on their own. They might even call up a professor and try to manage a better grade for their kid. A snowplow parent is the same but always ready to swoop in at a moment's notice, blast obstacles out of the way, and save kids from every potential harm or danger. They often work hard at securing extra advantages and boosting their child's chances of success ahead of others.

These types of parenting show up in many forms. These parents may write entire essays for the child, hire armies of tutors to keep grades up, and talk with sports coaches about getting more playing time. When you get right down to it, these types of parents care more deeply about their child's success than the child does. Just look at the news, where once-renowned public figures Felicity Huffman and Lori Loughlin were charged for fraudulently getting their children into college.

In an interview with *Huffington Post* in 2014, Huffman showed the amount of pressure she was feeling as a mom. A few years before her scandal, she had talked about how mothers live under an "amazing amount of pressure" on how their kids will turn out. "[W]hether they're gonna climb a tower and shoot people or go to Harvard might depend on how you handle this meltdown."[47] Apparently, the burnout had caught up with her.

By 2019, court documents show that Huffman, 56, was ordered to pay $30,000, perform up to 250 hours of community service, serve 14 days in prison, and endure one year of supervised release because she had, according to authorities, paid a college counselor to "correct wrong answers on her oldest daughter's SAT scores in 2017."[48] That pressure apparently did

---

47 Ryan Buxton, "Felicity Huffman Honestly Explains The 'Amazing Amount of Pressure' on Parents," Huffington Post, September 29, 2014, https://www.huffpost.com/entry/felicity-huffman-motherhood_n_5902674.
48 Kevin Breuninger, "Actress Felicity Huffman Sentenced to Two Weeks in Jail in College Admissions Cheating Case," CNBC, September 13, 2019, https://www.cnbc.com/2019/09/13/felicity-huffman-sentenced-in-college-admissions-cheating-case.html.

its worst on Huffman, and it could push anyone to make rash decisions as well. Something as big as fraud to something as small as never allowing your kids to have one single hiccup can have its consequences on them and, most importantly, on you.

Helicopter and snowplow parenting are side effects of a parent going all-in on their role as a mom or dad. It happens when our identity is tied up in being a mother or father. And for some reason, this seems to be much more likely to happen to women in our culture than to men. When people in the media talk about helicopter parents, they usually mean helicopter moms.

Helicopter moms have gone all-in on motherhood. They've started to see their kid's every success as a kind of parenting gold star and, therefore, an indicator of their own parental self-worth. Of course, we all feel good when our kids do well at something; that's only natural. But there's a fundamental difference between feeling good for *your child* and feeling good about *yourself*. When your children's wins or losses make you feel good or bad about yourself, it means you've got too many chips on your mom identity. You're in danger of going all-in, and you're likely to feel pressure to helicopter parent your kids.

Helicopter parenting is highly addictive because when it works, it makes you feel incredibly good about yourself; you saved the day. Your kid succeeded, thanks to you. Good job! For this reason, it's easy to justify. Some common reasons helicopter moms cite in defense of their actions include the following:

- I just want my kid to have all the resources they need to succeed.
- My kid couldn't do it without me; they don't have the capacity to realize the impact this will have on their lives!
- It's easier if I just do it for them anyway.
- My kid doesn't take initiative now, but they will if I can get them through this stage.
- My kid is too young or too big (or any other sort of excuse you need to get it done your way).

We understand the desire to see your kids fulfill their dreams. As moms, we want the world for our kids, of course. But when parents do this, it sends damaging messages.

If a parent is always handling difficult situations for their child, the child will internalize the message that they are not able to do things on their own. When a parent steps in to save a child by negotiating on their behalf, the child doesn't feel full ownership for their success. In the back of their mind, they have a nagging feeling that maybe they couldn't have done it without mom. Eventually, they may lack the confidence to speak up for themselves—since mom has always taken care of things for them.

Typically, the harder you work at something, the better it turns out. That's common sense. But the science reveals that with parenting, this isn't necessarily the case. Studies show that overparenting is just as detrimental to a child's anxiety and depression as underparenting.

Being the son or daughter of a helicopter parent might sound like a cakewalk—everything is taken care of! What an easy and stress-free life, right? But in reality, it can be a lot of responsibility for a kid to handle. For example, when you see your mother burst into tears because you didn't get the lead in the school play, you'll learn that it's up to *you* to make your mom happy. If you don't perform well, she'll be devastated. The child slowly gets the message that their actions are responsible for how mom feels. But this isn't fair. It's way too much pressure to put on a kid. A child absolutely cannot be responsible for an adult's feelings—kids are barely able to manage their own feelings most of the time! Imagine adding all of our inner anxiety into their little selves. Check, please!

Kids can certainly bring their parents plenty of happiness and joy. You shouldn't feel bad about feeling good for your kids. But the science is clear: relying *solely* on others to fill up your happiness bucket doesn't work.

> *"When you parent, it's crucial you realize you aren't raising a "mini me," but a spirit throbbing with its own signature. For this reason, it's important to separate who you are from who each of your children is. Children aren't ours to possess or own in any way. When we know this in the depths of our soul, we tailor our raising of them to their needs, rather than molding them to fit our needs."*
>
> —Shefali Tsabary, The Conscious Parent[49]

---

49 Shefali Tsabary, *The Conscious Parent: Transforming Ourselves, Empowering Our Children* (Vancouver, BC: Namaste, 2010).

When you find other ways to pursue purpose and meaning in your life that don't depend on your kids, it can actually feel like you're lifting a giant weight off your children's shoulders. They no longer have to be the only one responsible for your happiness. They are free to fail and make mistakes and do things differently than you expect without having to worry their actions might devastate you. They can focus on living their own lives, living and learning for their own purpose and development, and making decisions on how much they are willing to put at stake because they alone will have to pay the consequences should they fail.

It's not selfish as a mom to start taking time to pursue your own interests and passions. You're setting your children free from the burden of being your only source of fulfillment. The more avenues you have in your life to pursue your passions and do things that inspire you, the less pressure there is on your children to be perfect.

Of course, finding passions other than parenting isn't just good for your kids; it's good for you, too. When you allow someone else to be in charge of your happiness and satisfaction, you effectively give away your power to them. You relinquish control over your own inner state. Someone else now gets to decide how you feel about yourself. You are no longer the master of your thoughts and attitudes.

So, *stop it!* Stop giving away your power to your children.

If you rely on others to fill up your happiness bucket, it will never overflow. You will always be left wanting more. No one is a mind reader, and no one can give you exactly what you want—especially not your kids.

> *"Example isn't another way to teach. It's the only way to teach."*
> —Unknown

Overidentifying and overparenting can be crippling for our kids' development into healthy, functioning adults. You don't have to go all-in to be a successful mom. In fact, spreading your chips around in other areas might be the best strategy, and it isn't hard.

GETTING BACK TO NUMBER ONE

"To everything I have ever lost, thank you for setting me free"
—@farawaypoetry

Moms are busy. If you can find a mom who isn't struggling to get everything done on a daily basis, we want to meet her because she's a rare and mythical breed. Raising kids takes up all of your free time and energy and that's basically an undisputed fact. So how is it possible to spread your chips around and start branching out and pursuing other passions when you barely have a free minute to make yourself a cup of tea in the morning?

Back in school we learned about the properties of liquids, solids, and gases. Our chemistry teacher told us that a gas is unique because it expands to fill whatever container you put it in. Years later, we have found that parenting works the same way. It expands to fill however much time and energy you have available. *But it also shrinks if you decide you want to give it less space.*

When you start to give parenting a little bit less space in your life, you might find that you'll have a better relationship with your kids. This might sound contradictory, but it's true. Their mess-ups won't phase you as much because you'll have other things that also fulfill and center you.

An obvious example of this is having multiple kids. Your first child takes up all of your time and even keeps you up at night. But then, once you have two kids, you still parent them both, and it doesn't require 48 hours per day. You somehow get it all done in 24—because you have to. And then your third kid comes along, and you *still* manage everything in just 24 hours per day. You just find a way to make it all work. You get three times as much parenting done in the same amount of time because that's just what you have to do.

MY FIRST STEP, BY M

After I had my second baby girl and sleeping routines started to get a bit better and allow me to catch up on my rest, I knew that it was time to focus on getting back to me. Since I had two children so close together in age, I would do everything I possibly could to coordinate schedules, meals, naps, and whatever it took to have a snippet of free space.

I know many friends who in these free times prefer to try new kitchen recipes, perhaps look for decoration ideas on Pinterest, or simply take a well-deserved nap. And I get it. But although I do love naps, something inside of me since my daughters were very young told me that I had to take advantage of those few free spaces to do something for me.

That was how I decided to create a children's book. My two-year-old daughter was extremely picky with her food, and I thought it was a good idea to make a children's book in her honor about our dinner negotiations. My first obstacle with this idea was that I couldn't speak English yet, but I managed somehow to make sentences with simple rhymes. Then I got to the drawing board and, again, realized that this was not my forte. I went online, found a friendly Philippine artist offering her services in watercolor, and closed a very penny-saving deal. And finally, I had no idea how or where to sell such a book. Everything was completely new for me. So, while my girls enjoyed their daily naps, I investigated all the options I had available. I ended up teaching myself how Amazon Kindle worked and decided to sell the book in e-book format.

And that's how Picky Mimi *was born. Although the objective of this book was never an economic one (thank goodness, because it would have been a disaster), the fact that I could go on Amazon and see my book published there for my daughters to see and read reinforced my belief that our children need for us to be happy. They need to see us being more than their moms. My girls need me to have my own interests, fulfilled and interested in things in life outside of the home so that I can then push them to do the same. And that's just what this first attempt gave me.*

If the idea of spreading your chips around sounds like it's going to create more work, we get it. Self-help books like *The 5 AM Club* are great in theory, but getting up at 5 a.m. to add 20 minutes of meditation and other things to your day doesn't work for everyone—especially when you've been up all night with a fussy five-month-old. Concepts like time management are tricky to apply when you are busy putting out fires all day with babies or children. Instead of feeling uplifted and motivated, these books often leave us feeling kind of bad for not being able to follow through on all the pointers.

You can find lots of useful advice in the self-help and pop psychology books, but most of them are targeted toward people who have lots of time and space for change. Let's face it: a lot of these books are for young (male) professionals.

SELF-HELP, SELF-MADE, SELF-DROWNED, BY Z

I discovered the world of self-help with Rory Vaden's book Take the Stairs: 7 Steps to Achieving True Success. *I took it from my husband's nightstand and found it to be a very short and interesting read. I knew that the self-help genre existed, but I had never really sat down to read any. You could say I was a bit of a snob when it came to success and thought that people who wanted success simply had to work hard and do things right. But here I was working harder than ever as a mom, doing everything as best as I could—and yet, the feeling of success was nowhere to be found! I wondered where success was in motherhood. My corporate background showed me that if I organized myself well and did all tasks at hand, I would be good. But motherhood, I realized, was not a to-do list; it was something else.*

A bit after that, my third pregnancy ended up in miscarriage, and my husband saw me cry for an entire month every morning and every night. I had no idea how hard it would be to lose a child. I was completely thrown off by the incredible amount of pain I did not expect to feel for a life that I hadn't even held in my own arms! Again, I found a topic that was, like matrescence, not something that came up during your usual coffee convo with friends.

After a couple of weeks of my crying, he gave me a book. It was The Miracle Morning for Writers *by Hal Elrod. I was relieved that, apparently, there was an easy step-by-step formula to feeling a bit better. I just wanted the pain to stop, I quickly started to apply all the steps. I wanted to get myself back together, and these self-help books seemed to have a lot of answers. They would surely get me back into shape through reason and three steps, five steps, or 12 steps to success and happiness. The answers were written! Amen! For four months, I woke up every day at 5 a.m., did the steps, and wrote 2,000 words. The world was my oyster, and I felt like I could fly.*

But once I got pregnant again, waking up at 5 a.m. to get in all of my steps of silence, scribing, visualization, exercise, reading, and affirmations (Elrod calls these the lifesavers) went out the window. The vomiting started, and all I wanted to do was stay in bed to forget about another day of feeling horrible. Since this was not possible, I went into survival mode, and everything that had to do with living a successful life was put on hold. I loved doing Hal Elrod's lifesavers steps every morning—I even missed them—but I could barely stand up during the day, much less wake up at 5 a.m.

I found that motherhood comes with lots of ups and downs, and while these books are amazing, you do have to consider that you need some sort of physical and hormonal stability to get it done. And for me, in some moments of my motherhood, basic needs such as eating, sleeping, and showering had been set aside in order to care for a very small baby. So where were Elrod's lifesavers for moms?

What I did realize was that in the few months that I had been able to apply Elrod's lifesavers, I had recovered a beautiful and amazingly rewarding feeling of success. I had felt that I was giving my life everything it had. I was in a better mood with my kids, and my husband and I were able to enjoy going to the park with them again instead of stressing out that I was not getting any writing done. This all happened because I was dishing out those 2,000 words and my book was in the making. But I wondered, how can I continue to feel this success even in the moments when motherhood hits hard and leaves you with little to no room to take on all of your different areas? I realized that understanding what matrescence is and how it works does give you some sort of peace. It's not that I had lost my mind or my writing capacity; this was a phase, and seeing it as such, I could be more alert to getting back to me, step by step, little by little, no rush, and first and foremost, being compassionate with myself.

Navigating matrescence without becoming an all-in mom takes some effort, just as breaking any habit does. But it starts with something that won't take up any extra time in your day: a mindset shift. Kids are a big responsibility, but if you don't look out for yourself first, you'll never be able to operate at your best for everyone else. Spreading your chips around is important if you want to reconcile the identity collision and get away from being worn out.

Getting back to being the number one priority in your own life is not as drastic as it sounds. It's just about listening to yourself when you're uncomfortable or dissatisfied. Speaking your truth to your team members, be it your husband, your mom, a mental health professional, or even your babysitter or kid's teacher can allow you to process what's going on and get the answers you need faster. Acknowledging those moments when you are not happy in your role as a mom is a huge step forward. This can be extremely difficult, particularly if you are used to putting on a happy face for the world or getting things done 100 percent. However, it's a vital step to acknowledge your full emotions, even the negative ones.

Though this acknowledgment is a great step, we wanted to uncover some specific recommendations for how to avoid an out-of-proportion identity collision and sail through matrescence with ease. Because so little research has been done on this important life transition, we had to conduct a study for ourselves.

CHAPTER 6

The Happy Moms Study

"Even though on the surface it looked like I was 'all-in' as a mom, I had been resisting my motherhood and trying to escape it to find myself. But I didn't need to escape my children, or escape my role as mother, to solve my identity crisis. I needed to accept my children and my role as a mother—our interconnectedness—more deeply. To let it all in, but not at the expense of my own happiness."

—Leslie J. Davis

After going over all these issues again and again, we decided to do something about it. We had questions and we wanted answers. But we wanted answers that would really give us peace and sanity. No more secret recipe, no step-by-step program. We all know that we have to take better care of ourselves—we know it, but how do we apply it? We both found ourselves really enjoying and thriving in motherhood, but what were we doing right, and where had we gone wrong in the past? We wanted to share with clear facts how to get moving to a better us, to a better you, in the most stress-free way.

So, we grabbed our "lab coats" and called up a friend who could help us out. We'd like you to meet Bernardita; you can call her B. She is one of our good friends, also mom of four (a requirement for all contributors to this book, apparently), and she has a bachelor's in psychology and a master's in educational psychology and investigation. We asked if she would run a quick study for us—and she was on board before we even asked her to contribute. Over the next few weeks, she surveyed hundreds of women about their lives, behaviors, and attitudes. Then she crunched the numbers, and some surprising results started to emerge.

The first step to any study, B told us, is a literature review. That means we had to go back and read all the other studies and articles that had ever been published about the topics we wanted to research. *Wow. Talk about a lot of work.* We spent hours reading everything we could find online and at the local library about matrescence, identity development during motherhood, and achieving life balance for moms. As we conducted our review, five categories kept popping up as areas where moms should focus on spreading their chips: work, family, social, health, and mental wellness. Experts across multiple disciplines have honed in on these five spheres as important facets of a full, happy, and abundant life.

Based on this research, as well as our own ideas about matrescence, we surveyed 623 women. From there, we chose 100 participants to take part in a more in-depth study tracking their actual behavior for a couple of weeks. We asked them to fill out a weekly planner where they would spread their chips around on the five areas proposed. Below is an example of a filled-out weekly planner:

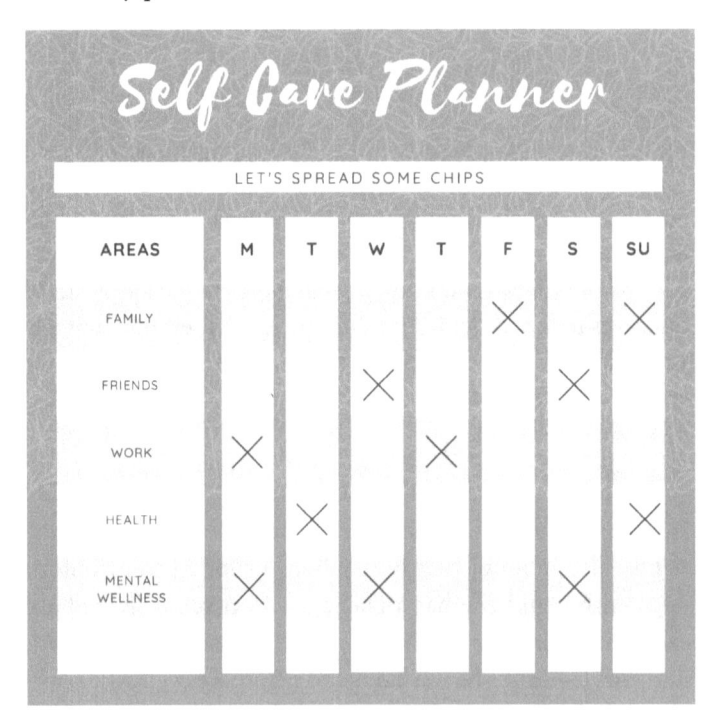

Self Care Planner

LET'S SPREAD SOME CHIPS

AREAS	M	T	W	T	F	S	SU
FAMILY					X		X
FRIENDS			X			X	
WORK	X			X			
HEALTH		X					X
MENTAL WELLNESS	X		X			X	

We give a quick summary of our findings here, and we explore these results in much greater detail in the following chapters.

Family: Women in our sample who reported being in stable marriages or partnerships were significantly more satisfied with their lives. This supports the notion that investing some time in maintaining your family relationships is a key driver of satisfaction and happiness. Strong relationships inspire and buffer us. By working hard to keep their intimate relationships healthy, happy moms reap huge rewards. Based on this data, we believe moms should devote energy each week to strengthening their relationships with each member of the family.

Social: Another thing we found was that women who socialized with at least one friend during the week, even virtually, rated their lives as more satisfying. Interestingly, it doesn't seem that increasing our socializing to 10 times per week gives much greater benefits than just a single session. We only found a benefit for one good session of socialization per week. It also appears that socializing works similarly to work and health: as long as you socialize at least once per week, you'll get the benefits.

Work: We found that women who reported participating in any sort of working activity at least once per week were more satisfied with their lives than were women who didn't. The study revealed no major difference in life satisfaction between women who worked full time, part time, or from home. This leads us to conclude that work doesn't have to be paid. Any position a woman can occupy outside of the house in which she can add value to an organization that she believes in, no matter how she does it, can have a positive impact on her identity. Also, once per week was enough for women in our study to see this benefit. This means whatever you choose to do for work doesn't need to require a large time commitment.

Health: Women in our study who reported exercising, even just once per week, were also more satisfied with their lives. From our data, it doesn't appear to make a difference what type of physical activity we get. What's important is to do it consistently, at least once per week. Additional activity beyond that is, of course, healthy and great, but we didn't see further improvement in life satisfaction past one exercise session per week. We suggest making this a high priority.

Mental Wellness: Another thing we found was that women who practiced any kind of spiritual activity were more satisfied with their lives than those who didn't. We learned that keeping a consistent spiritual practice of any sort reduces our stress, gives us hope and meaning, and helps us to trust ourselves when things get hard. Another interesting discovery was that the majority of women who practiced acts of gratitude, acts of kindness, and spirituality reported an increased satisfaction in life than those who didn't. We saw that small acts like these not only improve our general satisfaction in life, they also reduce stress, give us hope and meaning, and help us trust ourselves when the going gets tough.

These findings were consistent with the research that's already out there, which gave us more faith in our numbers. From our data, it appears that spreading our chips around to different areas of our identity, even just once a week, can significantly improve our satisfaction with life. Our results are directly linked to the statement "human beings are social creatures." From a psychological point of view, we know that humans need other people in order to survive and develop. Since the day we are born and throughout childhood, we need a person taking care of our physical health and nutrition, but above all, we need to have emotional support. A secure emotional environment that our stable relationships offer is our natural habitat no matter our geographical location. This is why we see in our study that the women who maintained stable family relations and those who took time to develop their friendships were the ones to confirm elevated satisfaction in life. Positive interaction with peers is a dopamine booster, and dopamine gives us feelings of pleasure and profound satisfaction.[50]

New technologies (such as FMRI, or functional magnetic resonance imaging) have allowed us to see our social need more concretely. Neuroscience has shown us that social relationships are deeply linked to the anatomy and biochemistry of our brain, affecting brain neuroplasticity. We need others to be able to discover ourselves, to evolve, and to be happy. This is why we have a social brain with a deep tribal instinct. We do better when we feel like we belong to a certain group. This could be at the base of our findings. Seeing that mothers who feel more satisfied with their lives to the extent that they have some type of job allows us to think that feeling that we're participating and collaborating with society, in some sense, makes us happier. Even science has shown us that social pain is felt at the brain level just like physical pain.

---

50 Sören Krach et al., "The Rewarding Nature of Social Interactions," Frontiers in Behavioral Neuroscience 4, no. 22 (May 28, 2010), https://doi.org/10.3389/fnbeh.2010.00022.

We live in a society that demands a lot from us, and as mothers, we often feel stressed. Maintaining physical exercise and meditation routines has been shown to decrease stress and allow us to better manage ourselves. This is why our results make sense to us when we see that those mothers who exercise physically and maintain some type of spiritual practice, such as meditating, feel more satisfied.

Importantly, our results suggest it won't necessarily require a huge time commitment to master matrescence; you just need to have a bit more mindfulness about how you are spending your time. The changes can be small, but you do really have to make them. Far too often we vow to make changes and then end up doing nothing at all. Once a week is all it takes to make a difference. But you have to actually do it once per week, and you have to keep at it.

THERE'S NOTHING WRONG WITH A LITTLE CHANGE

If someone doesn't want to change, they won't. Or as Jim Rohn once said, "I've discovered you can't change people, they can change themselves."[51] People have to want to change themselves; you can't do it for them. If you think anyone has ever changed you, think again. Perhaps you've been influenced by others, but ultimately it was always you who decided to make changes.

Change brings fear, but it also keeps us young and smart; every change we make in our routine means creating new neural connections in our brains. We encourage you to try it, and we are sure that you can do it! We'll help by providing a strategy to overcome fear of change and achieve what you want.

Amanda Gore is the CEO of The Joy Project and is one of the most popular experience-creating speakers in Australia and the US. She blends the principles of ancient wisdom with new research in modern science to wake people up to what really matters in life and at work. She proposes to follow these four steps:

1. Focus on what you want or need to change.

---

51 Jim Rohn, *7 Strategies for Wealth & Happiness: Power Ideas from America's Foremost Business Philosopher* (New York: Harmony, 1996).

2. Have awareness of the triggers that drive the behaviors you want to change.

3. Repeat for at least 21 days to create a habit.

4. Celebrate any change, big or small, along the way.[52]

Being forced to do happiness activities, the research shows, doesn't increase the happiness of participants afterward. However, when participants are able to choose which happiness-promoting activities they take part in, happiness does increase. This means being forced to exercise five days a week does not promote as much happiness as voluntarily exercising once per week. When we feel like we have more control over our choices and our lives, happiness and satisfaction trend upward.

Just as parents tell kids to try broccoli before they say they don't like it, we recommend trying out all five areas consciously for a while before you make any decisions about which ones are working best for you. Some things are acquired tastes and take time to develop. Certain activities may need to be tweaked to your preferences. Maybe meeting with a certain friend for coffee drags you down, but talking on the phone while walking lifts you up. Or you might find you enjoy group workout classes but not recreational sports.

As you read about each of the five categories, keep your mind open, and don't be afraid to start small. It's better to try something than to do nothing at all. There is no age limit for change; as long as you are motivated, you can always learn to do new things. This concept is another contribution of neuroscience. In addition to what was previously thought—that children are like sponges that can absorb a lot of new information and learn easily—we now know that adults are also capable of learning new information. It's all about staying motivated and being consistent in exercising the new habit.

You can start with what you know you do well, and this will give you the security you need to be able to move forward with the changes that cost you the most. There is nothing you cannot do, only challenges that you have not yet accomplished. Trust yourself; it is a matter of continuing to

---

52 "The Secret Formula for Change – You Need to FARC," Amanda Gore, accessed October 27, 2020, https://amandagore.com/the-secret-formula-for-change-you-need-to-farc/.

try and congratulating yourself for each small or great achievement that you accomplish. If you have setbacks, take them with humor; do not make it a drama, but check what happened, laugh at it, and take another turn with a new perspective. It's a matter of ingenuity, as when your own kids are learning to talk and walk. They aren't focused on what they can't do; they build on what they can and move from there!

TAKING CARE OF YOU FOR THEM

Remember that shifting some chips to the other areas of your life isn't selfish. It will, in fact, make you a better mom. When you aren't feeling 100 percent, how can you expect to be giving anything else your all?

One quote we stumbled upon in writing this book is from the late motivational speaker and life philosopher, Jim Rohn. Instead of "I'll take care of you if you take care of me," Rohn used to say, "I'll take care of *me* for *you* if you take care of *you* for *me*." At first this may sound a bit anti-romantic. After all, it sounds so much more romantic to fall in love and get swept away by someone. But maybe taking care of yourself for someone else is truly the most romantic and sexy thing there is. Maybe.

Stick with us here. By making this promise, you are, in effect, saying, "I will work hard, eat healthy, and take care of my own needs so that I am my best self for you." Contrary to what some dogmas may tell you, taking care of yourself is not a disservice to others. As our own survey showed, taking care of your needs is highly important and within your control. Looking to others to fill up your bucket puts an unfair burden on them. No one is going to be able to take care of you better than you. You know what you need and when you need it better than anyone.

Take a healthy diet, for example. You know that if you want to lose weight or eat healthier, you must have a balanced diet. The key here is exactly that word, balanced. You should eat your protein, carbs, grains, eggs, dairy, veggies, and fruit accordingly to get the health benefits you are looking for. Using this as a simile, your family area will probably be as important in your overall life satisfaction as proteins are to a healthy diet (sorry, veggies!), but you would never eat only proteins, right? You should add to your plate all the other components that make it well balanced. Same thing applies in your life. Add a little bit of socializing, work, spirituality, and health to your main course, and you will see the benefits of it.

The point of our study was to prove that life satisfaction comes from the combination of playing our chips on various areas of life at once. We wanted to prove that it's a life full of different activities that keeps us skipping and humming. In our study, 78 percent of the women were moms, but the results show that we should also pay attention to areas of their lives besides motherhood. From our study, we could officially conclude that levels of satisfaction in life could be predicted by being aware of healthy habits, conscious time with the family, social time, spiritual practice, and work.

We'll look at those areas more closely and see exactly what women need to do in each of these five categories to thrive during matrescence and beyond.

First up, family refocused.

CHAPTER 7

Family 101

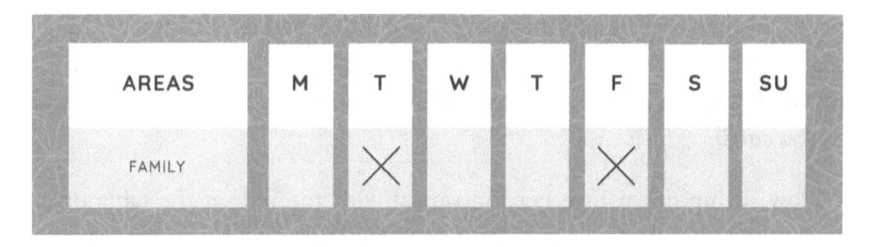

AREAS	M	T	W	T	F	S	SU
FAMILY		X			X		

"Notice when you're happy and know when you've got enough."
—Kurt Vonnegut, If This Isn't Nice, What Is?

It seems the more connected we get to our devices, the more disconnected we get with our loved ones. There's also a disconnection between our actions and the meaning behind them. We live in a whirlwind, being constantly stimulated all day long, and we're doing the same to our kids. We are filling their schedules up, but often we miss the purpose and meaning behind the activities. We need to bring purpose and love back to our daily actions.

In order to get more out of the time and energy we invest in our family, it's critical to become more conscious and aware of ourselves. Before we talk about our relationship with our kids, though, we need to look at the one we have with our partners.

BETTER TOGETHER

If you're a single parent, this section might not be relevant to you, and we won't be offended if you decide to skip down to the one on kids. But even if you're just seeing someone, you might find it useful.

Often after becoming a parent, it's easy for your romantic relationship to become transactional. You and your spouse see each other a lot, but it's always rushed and crazy, and you have only a small amount of attention available to exchange. On some level, you know that there is possibly no other relationship more important than the one you share with your partner. The two of you have forged an intimate and loving bond and are committed to raising kids together.

For most couples with kids, it's hard to find the right moments to fully enjoy the relationship. Before the kids arrived, you used to go on dates, cook meals together, have friends over, maybe travel a bit, attend spontaneous events ("Let's go to the movies tonight!"), and do all sorts of things together, just the two of you, just because. Back then, you could stay up for hours talking about anything and everything. No topic was too grand or too small.

Now sitting down together for a meal with the kids at the table or in the rocker has a timer on it. Your attention is focused on either how many spoonfuls you will get into his little mouth before he loses interest, or how many spoonfuls *you* will get into *your* mouth before he loses interest. Another fun fact is that although enjoyable at times, sitting at the family table with your partner can now come with each person's take on what proper manners are or discussions on parental feeding ideologies, such as negotiation ("OK, three more spoonfuls and you can have dessert") or ultimatums ("If you don't eat your food, you can't have dessert").

Then once the kids start getting older, you have the antenna issue, as we like to call it. It's all of those subjects that you used to be able to talk about with your partner in front of the kiddos when they were babies and incapable of understanding squat. But once their little brains start to grow and their little ears start to measure your tone of voice, they start to understand almost everything. Sometimes they will get what you're talking about, and other times they'll catch a phrase completely out of context and run with it. We're all about being honest with our kids about everything. But sometimes, at 6:30 p.m., you might want to steer clear of talking about issues such as world politics or if your mother-in-law made a good or bad decision, unless you are willing to receive lots of questions from your mini me for days on end.

As you can see, sitting at the dinner table might turn into a Navy SEAL boot camp. It's a matter of tactics, strategy, and team building, and, yes, you can put this on your CV, at least we think so. After awhile, you might feel like sitting down to eat with your partner and the kids has turned into part of the routine, such as brushing teeth and nighttime tuck-ins, almost like a check off of your to-do list. But it shouldn't be like this!

Also, if you both work, kids are around *all the time* when you are at home, leaving you and your partner with very little opportunity to be alone together. This makes couple moments extremely difficult to do. Being alone with your partner is important, however, because that is when you have a chance to focus on growing your relationship. But with kids in the picture, there are very few opportunities to achieve this in a nonstressful and spontaneous way. These moments are rare but necessary, and they really should become part of your weekly schedule.

A 2004 University of North Carolina study of "relative happy, non-distressed couples" showed that couples who practiced mindfulness saw improvements in their relationship happiness. In addition, they experienced healthier levels of "relationship stress, stress coping efficacy, and overall stress."[53]

Practicing mindfulness with your partner doesn't necessarily mean lighting candles and gazing into his or her eyes while holding hands on a beach and listening to each other's beating hearts. It's simply taking a second to check in on your other half. Ask them how they're doing and find out if they need to talk about something—opening up in general is healthy. Mindfulness is about complimenting your partner genuinely whenever you can.

> "We now know that love is, in actuality, the pinnacle of evolution, the most compelling survival mechanism of the human species. Not because it induces us to mate and reproduce. We do manage to mate without love! But because love drives us to bond emotionally with a precious few others who offer us safe haven from the storms of life. Love is our bulwark, designed to provide emotional protection so we can cope with the ups and downs of existence. This drive to emotionally attach—to find someone to

---

[53] James W. Carson et al., "Mindfulness-based relationship enhancement," *Behavior Therapy* 35, no. 3 (2004): 471–494.

> *whom we can turn and say 'Hold me tight'—is wired into our genes and our bodies. It is as basic to life, health, and happiness as the drives for food, shelter, or sex. We need emotional attachments with a few irreplaceable others to be physically and mentally healthy—to survive."*
>
> —Sue Johnson, Hold Me Tight: Seven Conversations for a Lifetime of Love[54]

Usually the main reason romantic partnerships suffer is that both parents are just so damn busy. When life reaches a busyness breaking point, it is easy to resort to going-through-the-motions mode. It can feel like your lives are running you instead of you running your lives. Pretty soon it's the automatic routines that are holding everything and everybody in the family together. You're in the same house, taking care of the same kids, eating the same food, walking the same dog but not really connecting in meaningful ways.

Yes, you and your beloved spend countless hours *together* every week, but precious few minutes *alone together* in an environment where you can truly talk and connect. You need to make time for each other. And mom, the first effort needs to come from you. Why? Because you're reading this book, and you're searching for something. And the first step to fixing or making something better must always start with us, the ones needing that change or improvement. Stop waiting and expecting the other person to make changes so that you get what you want. Get it yourself.

Find some alone time with your partner. This doesn't have to be a huge ordeal where you leave the house, have a fancy dinner, and spend a lot of money. It could be putting down your phones one hour before bed each night. Or you could feed the kids early one night and open a bottle of wine on the porch. Find time to get the conversation going.

If you want to go out, hire a babysitter or ask your parents to watch the kids for an hour once every week or two. Maybe ask them for a *few* hours so you can catch dinner and a movie. And again, turn the phones off during this time. Just be together. This will keep you as alert as possible to really take in the other person.

---

54 Sue Johnson, *Hold Me Tight: Seven Conversations for a Lifetime of Love* (New York: Little, Brown Spark, 2008).

Other ideas in earlier hours of the day could be instituting quiet time, where your kids have to limit themselves to individual silent activities, such as reading a book, playing with dolls, doing a puzzle, or coloring. Set a timer to go off when quiet time is over. Explain that it's important for everyone to practice having time to be quiet and independent for part of the day. You can further explain that parents need to have some quiet time to be alone together if you think your kids will understand that.

> *"It is not a lack of love, but a lack of friendship that makes unhappy marriages."*
> —Friedrich Nietzsche

MOM AND DAD TIME, BY Z

My kid's school had a family therapist give a chat about how to help your children grow up to be brave or something like that, and as part of her presentation she mentioned something I had never heard was a real thing. She talked about "Mom and Dad time."

She said it was important for kids to understand the concept of how Mom and Dad happily invest their time during the day to be with them, care for them, play with them, etc., but at one point, usually at night, it becomes Mom and Dad time. She said that this gives kids a sense of respect for other people's time and lives, and it would also help them value their time with us more. I remember that this blew my mind, because up until then, every time my husband and I had left the kids with a babysitter (we had two toddlers and a very small baby then), we would literally sneak out. We would do bedtime as usual. I would change into my PJs like it was a regular night, I would read them their bedtime stories, pray a bit, and leave the room.

Once they were asleep, I would change into my dinner clothes, shoes in hand, let the babysitter in, sit her down in front of the TV, leave her some instructions and snacks, and literally run. My kids never saw a single babysitter at night for years. They were great first-hour sleepers. I would leave and know that for at least three to four hours, the chances of them waking up were low.

We always felt like two teenagers, running out into the night, praying for the kids to not wake up. Then one night, it happened. I remember getting the call at a restaurant, halfway through a meal that had been planned for weeks. The babysitter could not put one of my kids down to sleep again and was not able to comfort the child at all. She sounded nervous, so I ran home even more nervous than the both of them. I felt like I had been caught, and it felt terrible.

After I attended that talk, we decided to sit down with the kids and talk to them about how Mom and Dad need *to be together alone, in order to be* better *parents for them. My second was around four and did not like the plan, but after a couple of trials he finally felt comfortable with the idea. It immediately dropped our anxiety levels 50 percent every time we took a moment for ourselves after that. We still do their entire nighttime routine with them that involves bath time, PJs, dinner, brushing teeth, reading a couple of books together, praying, and listening to their favorite nighttime song on Spotify, but we are very open at the dinner table about Mom and Dad's dinner plans after they get in bed. Sometimes I get dressed up before their bedtime, and the conversation starts naturally. "Why are you wearing that? Where are you going?" my five-year-old might ask. And I very coolly respond (inside I'm praying for a calm reaction), "We have dinner with friends tonight." Should a tantrum occur, my speech is always ready to go: "Mom and Dad have been with you guys all day, and we had a great time! But now Mommy and Daddy need time to be together, to talk about all of the fun things we can plan with you guys tomorrow (it's a win-win situation, kid), and now it's your time to go to sleep."*

Spend your quiet time alone with your partner on the porch or in the basement. Drink a glass of wine or try a new kombucha flavor together. Try to keep it simple and fun. Maybe share something one of you read that you found interesting, or maybe one of you is struggling with something and you need someone to brainstorm with safely. You can have a conversation or just sit in silence, looking out onto your street or backyard or at a view of the city. No screens are allowed so that nothing that can take attention away from just being with each other. Make it a routine and make it a priority. The first time you try this, it might feel forced or phony. But that's OK. Keep going. Over time, it should get easier to switch over to adult conversation, and interruptions from kids should become fewer as you enforce the rules.

This is just a starting point but an important one. If you don't block out the time, it just won't happen. For most things in your life, especially the important ones, you must schedule them. You have to write them on your agenda and set a reminder on your phone. If you wait for the end of the day to squeeze this in during the final hour before bed, you'll end up too exhausted to really focus on each other on a deep level. Get deliberate about your quality couple time. When you create time consciously, it has a different character than when you just stumble along and take what you can get.

One hour may not sound like a lot of time, but it can feel like an eternity when you're fully present with each other and focused on nothing else except just being together and connecting. It's not the amount of time that matters; it's being fully invested in that time. This is easiest when you specifically set the time aside and dedicate it to your relationship. It's also easier when you don't have any distractions like a project to work on together, a meal to consume, or chore to get done. Just be together and talk about whatever comes up or sit in silence. The only rule is you can't talk about the kids! Only adult conversation topics are allowed.

As you incorporate more of this type of conscious togetherness into your relationship, you can, of course, move up to spending longer periods of time alone together. But try to find ways to bring that same level of absolute presence to every session.

THE COAST IS CLEAR, BY M

When my kids were babies, we couldn't afford a babysitter, had no family around, and between diaper changes and breastfeeding, time was scarce. So, my husband and I started to work on our kids' routine just a little bit harder, to perfect it to the point where we knew we would have our own quiet, private weekend lunches together at our own dinner table without kids around. We would take the girls outside during the morning, give them a good amount of physical activity, feed them their lunch, and secure our one to two hours of their nap time to be together and talk.

It took us a good couple of years to be able to hire a babysitter, but just knowing that we could both look forward to that Saturday lunch together would change my week. I knew that I could count on those moments, and by the time we were able to afford a babysitter, we started to implement the same practice with long walks together and dinner at the local restaurant with cost-friendly menus. Most of our family goals and a lot of what we have accomplished up to date was brainstormed and thought out during those small moments. It gave us the chance to not only see ourselves as a great team as parents, but as a great team at running our lives and our dreams.

ESCAPE FROM THE ISLAND, BY Z

Before I had kids, I knew a married couple who went on an overnight getaway together once every month, leaving their three children at home in the care of a grandma. I was young and very far away from understanding the realities of married life with kids. This idea seemed strange and even expensive to me. I earned a small salary at the time, and the numbers simply didn't add up. Why would someone pay an entire rent on a house and then go sleep in their same neighborhood, just 10 blocks away? I trusted they had good reason, but I didn't understand how two people who already lived together needed to be together outside of their home. "Isn't it the same thing?" I wondered.

Now, with four kids and 10 years of marriage, I can say, hands down, they were brilliant. This couple was deliberately carving out time to focus on each other and their relationship without distraction. They were prioritizing conscious togetherness.

Years later, when my husband was studying for his Executive MBA at Kellogg School of Management, he would have his classes at the Coral Gables Campus here in Miami. Every month, he would leave from Thursday to Sunday, and he would bunk up in the hotel next to the school like the rest of his cohorts. Sometimes, maybe Friday or Saturday late afternoon, he would show up at home to be with us. The first year, I was pregnant with my fourth so his coming back and helping out with the kids was very much appreciated. But the second year, I decided to use those hours differently. Instead of having him over to help out, now that the kids were a bit bigger, I used those hours to go visit him. I almost felt like a college kid visiting my boyfriend's dorm. We would go out and have dinner from the hotel and just enjoy our presence, our time, with no rush. It felt amazing.

And that's how we started to pay attention to finding our own little moments throughout the year. Sometimes we're so tired that we barely talk during dinner. But just enjoying the silence and each other goes a long way. If we had our family close by, maybe I would find a way to have the kids sleep over at my parents' house. But since we are on our own, I made it a point to find a trusty auntie-like babysitter who can make the kids feel at home when I'm out for 14 hours.

Another plus I discovered was being able to dress up a little bit. Putting on nice earrings knowing they won't be yanked from my earlobe is nice! Wearing a nice dress knowing it won't get spit or vomit on it is very different from wearing clothes that I'm OK with having a little bit of color variation, if you know what I mean.

By taking time for your relationship, you are showing your kids that marriage or adult relationships are important and require significant and visual effort. Depending on your kids' age, you will need more or less. We find that when the kids are young, the housework is demanding, and waiting for them to go off to college is a bit too late. The work has to start now, and by work we mean getting the babysitter booked, picking out your nice clothes, and simply allowing yourself to relax every so often. It will take a bit of planning and thinking outside the box. We know it might not be easy, but if you put your mind to it, we're sure you'll find a place in your schedule.

You and your partner made it this far because you both put in the work to build your relationship. Having kids may complicate things, but it shouldn't detract from the quality of the time you spend together.

Going through the motions of intimacy (asking about each other's day, talking about the kids) is different than meaningfully connecting, and it feels shallow. Being mindful and present about your intimate relationship will take practice, but slowly chipping away at it will pay dividends in the quality of your partnership and in the example you are setting for your kids. Plus, it's a great excuse to relax for a while.

So, go ahead, throw some chips at this area and conquer that lost territory. It's never too late.

THE RUSH TO NOWHERE

Even before your kids were born, your life has been essentially revolving around those little people nonstop. Wouldn't it be great if you could achieve an even greater impact during the hours you are already spending with your kids? You might even be able to cut those hours down a bit so you can ultimately focus more time on the other parts of yourself. It's the good ol' quality versus quantity effect again. Most importantly, we want to talk about what you can do to start feeling a greater sense of purpose and fulfillment from the same hours you're already spending with your children. We want to increase your parenting efficiency.

The answer isn't that you need to start filling your hours with more grand, exciting, and fabulous parenting adventures. This isn't about throwing a party, visiting the zoo, and planning a trip to Disneyland. Our recommendations are actually a lot more mundane than all of that. This is more about the things you're already doing right now. It's about the family dinners, the bedtime routines, and the afternoon walks. We're just going to talk about how to get more out of them.

IT'S IN THE LITTLE THINGS, BY Z

I was 23 years old when I lost my mom to cancer. She was my everything, my home, my true companion. We had moved around so much because of my dad's job, losing mom was almost like losing home. I thought it was just me until I started to talk to other people in mourning. I realized that often when you lose someone close, the things you miss most are the small, daily details, or "the usual."

I realized that in a rush to keep my kids entertained and stimulated all the time, I was doing a lot of extra, unnecessary things. For instance, I started to get a yearly pass to the science museum. I would drive for miles and take them to see the exhibits on gravity and the fun demonstrations with fire and slime. But I saw that what I missed most about my own mom was simply being with her, seeing her laugh, and feeling her hands. She was a pianist, and I would spend hours playing with her hands and looking at them, turning her rings around and around on her soft, beautiful fingers. She had the most delicate and soft hands in the world. I wanted my kids to have more of those types of casual, intimate memories with me, so I started to sit down with my kids on the mat in their room with no phone or TV to distract us.

I had always read books to my kids every night, but after three years of parenting, the routine was starting to get a bit stale. To make things worse, I was pregnant with my third child and was feeling tired and heavy. Every night sitting on the floor started to get harder, I became more uncomfortable, and I started to rush through the books to get them done and over with. So, I broke the bedtime routine during my pregnancies and let them lie in my own bed, with my feet up on a couple of cushions, and read them their books. Then my husband would take them to their beds and tuck them in. That's when I realized they deserved my full attention for 10 or 20 minutes. Soon, storytelling became a very special time. When I sat on the edge of the bed and opened up a book, something would click in my kids, peace would settle over the room, and love would fill up the air.

Don't underestimate the power of the little stuff. The small mundane moments are what motherhood is really about, not the big flashy stuff. But most of the time, we aren't fully invested in these small, habitual interactions. When we're burnt-out from a long day or busy thinking about our to-do list for the coming week, we can fail to be completely present.

When we focus on the outcomes for our kids, the process becomes less important. When we fail to see the value of the process is when our voices start to get a little bit louder, our nerves get a little bit crispier, and we feel that the whole planet is going to blow up if that kid doesn't get to soccer practice on time. Our kids will remember the emotional environment over whether we did everything for them to get it right.

The solution isn't to take your kids on more trips to the science museum or to buy them more toys. The solution is to simply become more mindful, conscious, and present.

> *"Become silent in your children's presence, free yourself of all distractions, and attune yourself to them in a state of curiosity and delight."*
> —Dr. Shefali Tsabary[55]

THE GREATEST GIFT, BY M

One morning last summer, a friend of mine shared a PDF called "Summer Activities for Your Kids" in our mom group chat. It was full of Pinterest-inspired, impossible-to-do activities, nature discovery adventures, and all-day trips. I took a look at the list and nothing really grabbed my attention. It all seemed to involve long hours in the hot sun, a road trip, or an arsenal of new arts and crafts supplies. The options just didn't sound particularly appealing to me. But in the chat, my friends went crazy with responses.

"What great ideas," one friend replied. "I'm going to take my kids to the zoo! If anyone wants to join, let me know." In this Florida summer heat? No, thanks.

"My daughter is super bored," said another friend. "I'm going to take her on the train ride up to Palm Beach!" Honestly, that sounded exhausting to me.

---

55 Tsabary, *The Conscious Parent*.

As the messages poured in, I started to feel exhausted and a little anxious. I handed my phone over to my oldest daughter and asked her to look over the activities list and see what caught her eye. "Mom, we don't really need any of these things," she said. "We're just fine here with you, and I have the best activity in the world: playing with my two sisters and little brother." My jaw dropped and my heart filled up. I realized she was absolutely right.

Our kids don't need the over-the-top gifts, vacations, or playdates. They just need our undivided attention.

MINDFUL PARENTING

Mindful parenting is all the rage right now. If you want your kid to be aware of his or her actions and feelings, this will require an adult to be aware of his or her own actions and feelings. Conscious and aware parents are what kids need. Period.

We can't claim credit for this marvelous insight. Researchers have been onto this important tidbit for years now. In a 2016 study, parents who practiced mindfulness ended up having a greater number of positive interactions with their child.[56] Additionally, the children of more mindful parents exhibited fewer behavioral problems and increased emotional literacy as compared to a control group. Mom-child mindfulness studies in other countries from all over the world have demonstrated similar results. All types of parent-child interactions show improvement with mindfulness practice.

Mindfulness is one of the simplest known solutions for increasing fulfillment in parenting. It's a buzzword that gets thrown around a lot these days, usually in the context of meditation. If you read many self-help books, you might have noticed that they usually have a chapter on the benefits of mindfulness meditation, urging you to start meditating.

This isn't one of those books.

If you want to sit around in the lotus position, that's great. But we think it's important to talk about mindfulness on a larger scale. Becoming more

---

[56] Lisa M. May et al, "Parenting an Early Adolescent: A Pilot Study Examining Neural and Relationship Quality Changes of a Mindfulness Intervention," *Mindfulness* 7 (2016): 1203–1213, https://doi.org/10.1007/s12671-016-0563-3.

conscious and deliberate in your daily interactions with your children can make a huge difference in how you connect and grow together as a family. Instead of trying to plan lots of extraordinary activities and trips, moms can simply step back from the pressure to give their kids everything and focus on what kids really need the most: your full, undivided attention. In fact, it's what we all want the most from each other; kids are no different.

Rather than running through your to-do list in your head and living in a constant state of distraction, you can choose to be fully present with your children. You can consciously interact with them instead of trying to speed things up and move on to the next task. When other thoughts beyond the things you are doing in the current moment slip into your mind, simply bring yourself back to the present moment.

Let's say you're on a walk in the park with your four-year-old, chatting away with each other, when a thought wanders in about being on time for a haircut later. Instead of ruminating on it, acknowledge it. Sometimes it helps to actually say things out loud: "Ah yes, I've got a haircut later. Thanks for reminding me." And then return to the present.

Returning to the present may sound difficult, but you can usually achieve it by tuning into the sights, sounds, and feelings in front of you and around you. Reengage with it all. If you're in the park, for example, maybe you can notice the sound of the birds, make eye contact with your child, or squeeze a small hand to bring yourself back to the present. The great thing about practicing mindfulness and turning on your senses in the presence of your children is that for them, this world is new and exciting. Maybe you've been to the same park a thousand times, but with your kids, you can discover it anew, finding new details, meeting new people, and laughing at new jokes. Go ahead, be a kid with them for a little while. Step into their awe of the world, and you'll find yourself slipping into a deep state of "being together."

Being mindful with your child also means acknowledging when things are hard or when you become upset. For example, if our kid is dragging his feet to get out the door in the morning, we often don't say anything about it, and then we end up mumbling under our breath how unbelievably annoying he's behaving during the entire car ride. Instead, you can acknowledge that you are angry and say, "Being late makes me feel really frustrated and stressed out." Simply labeling emotions can help to stop them from controlling your mind. Once you admit how you are feeling and experience the anger or sadness or frustration, you can move on from it.

This can also lead to a productive discussion with your child about tardiness. "I'm feeling frustrated because I'm not sure we will be on time for school," you could say. "If we are not on time for that, then I might be late for my own meeting. Other people can get upset when you are late because you already promised to be on time. Arriving late is disrespectful to other people, and I like to always treat others with respect." Putting words to how you feel is the basis for effective human interaction.

Again, doing this sort of thing takes practice. You probably won't get it perfect the first time around—you're human after all! But keep pushing through. To keep it up on a daily basis, you will have to find a way to remind yourself about it.

BREATHE IN, BREATHE OUT, BY Z

After reading a few books on the power of mindfulness, I was excited to get started. The data was right there in black and white. The results were in. Mindfulness was the answer to all my prayers, and so I started to practice it. I woke up early in the morning, didn't look at my phone, drank a long glass of water, set an intention of love for the day, walked into the kitchen, and put on some soft music. I kneeled and greeted my babies with hugs and kisses and started passing warm toast around. Beautiful. Namaste. I got this.

A couple of seconds later, two of the young ones got out of their seats and started to fight over who would get to pull the marmalade out of the fridge. That's when I saw the glass jar of marmalade fly across the room in slow motion and crash against the floor, shattering into a thousand pieces, and a deep roar came flying out of my vocal cords. Namaste was out the window. My mindfulness capacity was depleted.

As I knelt to the floor, cursing and mumbling in my head, I realized this mindfulness thing was going to be a bit harder to keep up than I'd imagined at first. I was starting to see why they say it's something you practice, not something you do.

I started to put little notes everywhere to remind myself to be present. I put notes in the car, bathroom, kitchen, shower, and on top of the TV. The notes all had just one word: Focus. I even stuck one of these notes to the back of my phone with tape. Every time I see it, I get a little Pavlovian reaction and am jolted back into a mindful state. I still have times where mindfulness gets thrown out the window, but I have a system in place to center myself.

We recommend trying to implement more mindfulness into your own parenting. When your day is full of activities, it's easy to get distracted. Try writing FOCUS into your daily schedule. Put BREATHE into your Google calendar, and shoot yourself a notification from time to time. It will help a lot. Try it for a few weeks to see if you notice any differences.

Mindfulness provides numerous benefits. First, you'll experience more positive interactions with your child. Also, your child will demonstrate better behavior and greater emotional regulation. When you approach parenting from a more present place, you'll notice a higher quality of interactions. And this is especially important to master when you're working to shift some of your chips away from your mom role and toward other aspects of your life.

CHAPTER 8

Friends

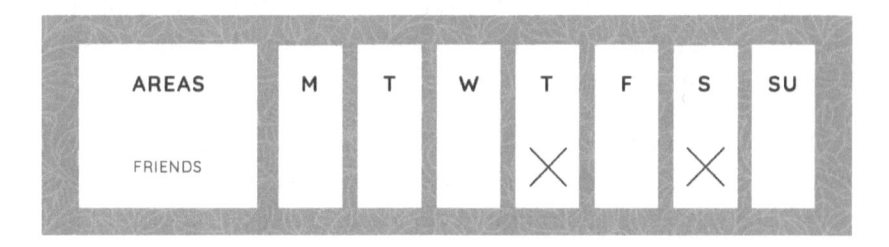

AREAS	M	T	W	T	F	S	SU
FRIENDS					X		X

> *"Among all worldly things there is nothing which seems worthy to be preferred to friendship...It is what brings us the greatest delight, to such an extent that all that pleases is changed to weariness when friends are absent."*
>
> —St. Thomas Aquinas

In a viral 2015 TED Talk on the meaning of life, Dr. Robert Waldinger, the director of the Harvard Study of Adult Development, said that "... good relationships keep us happier and healthier." This ongoing Harvard study is considered one of the world's longest studies of adult life ever conducted, having begun in 1938 during the Great Depression. "Our study has shown that the people who fared the best were the people who leaned into relationships: with family, with friends, and with community," Waldinger said.[57]

Being a mom can get lonely. Sure, you may have a spouse and there are

---

[57] Robert Waldinger, "What makes a good life? Lessons from the longest study on happiness," TED, recorded November 2015, https://www.ted.com/talks/robert_waldinger_what_makes_a_good_life_lessons_from_the_longest_study_on_happiness/transcript?language=en.

kids around 24/7 clamoring for your time and attention, but your spouse is often tired after a long day and wants to just zone out. Also, there's a huge difference between the types of interactions you can have with small kids and the types of interactions you can have with other adults. You just can't connect with your kids about the deep issues in life (nor do you want to when they are so young). We all need some friends who we can share our parenting struggles with, ask for advice, or laugh with at references from *Friends*, *Seinfeld*, and *Sex in the City*.

The sheer number of feelings a mom can have during a single day is almost unreal. You can jump from joy to fear to anger in less than an hour. This emotional roller coaster can become much more enjoyable simply by sharing it with friends. Feeling like you're not the only one going through the steps of learning how to care for children can make a huge positive impact on your self-esteem.

We all know it's important to maintain friendships outside of the home. We feel great on those rare occasions when we do get to spend an evening socializing with other adults instead of picking Play-Doh out of someone's hair. When these grown-up playdates end, we often find ourselves saying things like, "Wow, we should really do this more often," and, "It's been way too long since the last time we did something like that."

Then why is that when we become parents, our social life gets so diminished? One study on loneliness surveyed 2,000 parents and found the majority (68 percent) felt cut off from friends, colleagues, and family after the birth of a child. Common reasons for this feeling of isolation included lack of money and the inability to leave the house.[58]

Here are a few limiting thoughts we've found ourselves having about our social lives:

- "I'm just so tired at night, I couldn't possibly get out of the house once they fall asleep."
- "This is just temporary because they're little. Once they grow up, I'll have plenty of time for my friends."
- "My kids need me at the house just in case."

---

58 Kawther Alfasi, "The Loneliness of Early Parenthood," *The Atlantic*, February 5, 2020, https://www.theatlantic.com/family/archive/2020/02/loneliness-early-parenthood-mothers-estrange-friendships/606100/.

- "My husband would never stay alone with the kids while I'm having a night out with the girls."

Do any of those sound familiar? Maybe you have some different ones, or perhaps you have a rich social life, and this isn't a problem for you. But if you know a friend who never seems to be able to find the time, reach out and make her read this.

Research suggests motherhood can be particularly isolating. One survey of 2,025 new mothers found 54 percent admitted to feeling friendless after giving birth.[59] Suddenly you and your friends can't go to the same places you used to go to together, and your schedules are completely out of sync. Besides, you might not feel great either, or you probably need to catch up on some sleep now that you've got the little ones around. Sometimes the people you used to find entertaining lose their magic and you might start to drift apart.

Why is it so easy to find ourselves always putting family first, even though we know friends are important, too? It goes back to the splurge mentality in the mom guilt arena. As moms, we are conditioned to think of anything we do purely for ourselves as being a splurge, whereas the things we do for our family are seen as simply part of our duties. When we think this way, it's no wonder we rarely find time to socialize with other adults.

As moms, we push our own social lives to the side and vow to pick them back up when the kids get older and don't need us so much. We tell ourselves that maybe once the kids leave the house and head to college we'll get back to having friends because then we'll have more time and energy. But as we gradually give up our social lives, we're actually shifting more of our chips over to our mom identity. This makes us feel even worse accepting social invitations in the future, so we compensate by pushing our social life even further to the side until soon we don't have one at all. It's a vicious cycle.

Parenthood causes social distancing in our lives. A survey conducted during the coronavirus quarantine found that 45 percent of adults felt the pandemic affected their mental health, with 19 percent saying it had

---

59 Alfasi, "The Loneliness of Parenthood."

a major impact.[60] In a review, researchers evaluated 24 studies looking at the psychological outcomes for people who were quarantined during outbreaks of SARS, H1N1 flu, Ebola, and other infectious diseases that have occurred since the early 2000s. Many quarantined individuals experienced both short- and long-term mental health problems, including stress, insomnia, emotional exhaustion, and substance abuse.[61] We know it's not good to be isolated. But the strange thing is that when we become moms, we willingly isolate ourselves from social contact with other adults, cutting ourselves off from the possibility of meaningful friendships.

Historically, women were part of a tribe. Our ancient ancestors evolved in small groups and villages where social interaction was a constant part of daily life. Anthropological studies of hunter-gatherer civilizations indicate that early humans likely spent just 15-20 hours per week gathering food, and the rest of their time was devoted to playing, laughing, dancing, and talking with small groups of tribemates. Kids formed large groups and entertained themselves in those days, with the oldest children looking after the younger ones. This left parents with the vast majority of their time free to communicate with other adults.[62]

Tribe size averaged about 150 members, but it isn't likely that each member socialized equally with all other members. It's probably safe to say that early humans seem to have lived in large social groups of around 50 friends and extended family members. They likely communicated with nearly everyone in their social circle at least once per day.

Compare this to the typical mom today. The modern mom might chat with another parent as she drops her child off for a playdate. But often, these are friends of convenience rather than friends she's consciously chosen for herself. She may or may not feel a true sense of connection with

---

60 Joel Achenbach, "Coronavirus is harming the mental health of tens of millions of people in the U.S., new poll finds," The Washington Post, April 2, 2020, https://www.washingtonpost.com/health/coronavirus-is-harming-the-mental-health-of-tens-of-millions-of-people-in-us-new-poll-finds/2020/04/02/565e6744-74ee-11ea-85cb-8670579b863d_story.html.
61 Sören Krach et al., "The Rewarding Nature of Social Interactions," Frontiers in Behavioral Neuroscience 4, no. 22 (May 28, 2010), https://doi.org/10.3389/fnbeh.2010.00022.
62 Michaeleen Doucleff, "Are Hunter-Gatherers the Happiest Humans to Inhabit Earth?" NPR, October 1, 2017, https://www.npr.org/sections/goatsandsoda/2017/10/01/551018759/are-hunter-gatherers-the-happiest-humans-to-inhabit-earth.

them. Similarly, the modern mom may have a talk with her child's music instructor, coach, schoolteacher, and dentist. But these relationships all center around the child, not around the two adults who are actually having the conversation. If she works, this mom might have some acquaintances at the office. But most conversations there will revolve around work projects and office gossip. Work relationships can be highly fulfilling, and we absolutely encourage moms to work, but these workplace discussions don't take the place of social friendships.

I'LL HAVE A MEDIUM LATTE, BY Z

I am a huge homebody. I like going to sleep super early and waking up early. I love seeing my friends during the day and seeing them at night. I've always been the one that has a nice time during parties and weddings until I start to smell the dew on the grass that signals we are getting close to midnight or even past it. I automatically start wanting to head home like a horse walking back to its post. Motherhood has made me even more of a Cinderella. My precious firstborn has had the habit of waking up to greet Mr. Sun at 6 a.m. since the day she was born. Cutie.

But I yearned to be with my friends, talk about our lives, and connect with other people outside of my house and my kids' teachers during pick-up time. I feel a need to really sit down and see how my friends are doing, how they're feeling, maybe even process stuff that happens in my life, or talk about something that I've read or have been thinking about that I found interesting. But just talking at a park while your kids play can be tricky. First you have to check for antennas, aka your own kids. Then you have to be able to keep your train of thought while prying open someone's mouth to take out the grasshopper that should not be there.

One day during a vacation with a friend and her family, I started talking to my mom's friend about something. The conversation got deep, but we were both in the water with our kids floating and splashing around. It began to rain, so we rushed them inside, dried them off, and put together something for the kiddos to eat. Once they were finished eating, we washed their hands and handed out crayons and papers for them to draw while the rain continued to pour down outside. My friend and I were cleaning up in the kitchen and I continued our deep conversation right where I had left off. We talked and talked until someone needed a diaper change. I went upstairs, got the diaper and wipes, headed down, picked up the baby, cleaned his buttocks, fixed him a bottle, and went into his room to put him down for a nap. Twenty minutes later I walked out and found my friend looking at her cell phone while the older ones were watching TV. So, I picked up our convo again where it had been left off. That night we had dinner with our husbands on the porch, and we talked about other things.

The next day we were both back in the water with the kids. I made a reference to what we were talking about, almost picking up exactly where we had been last afternoon, and my friend started laughing. She said, "I find it fascinating that you have developed the capacity to have an entire conversation with a thousand interruptions. It's like listening to a book on Audible when I go out for a run!" I laughed as well and thought, Well, maybe this isn't normal but, hey, here I am making lemonade with my lemons!

I like to talk; I like to process things out loud; I like to hear feedback. I bless my friends and their points of views; I feel rich because I have them in my life. And I know that if I put them in the freezer and don't connect with them until motherhood gets less demanding, then I'm not giving myself the chance to connect with myself and enjoy the gift of their friendship. So, yes, I take our conversations seriously enough to not let a diaper change or a meal prep get in the way. This said, I did realize the amount of work I had to put in mentally to keep the hour-and-a-half conversation going over a period of 15 hours. I decided, then, to schedule in seeing my friends during the day. I'm much more lucid and myself during the morning. I know that one good hour of talking over coffee each week makes me feel alive and makes me connect with myself, even if we're talking about what the other person is going through or wants to say. Just listening to or being heard by a good friend can make wonders in my life. So, I stick to it—for everyone's sake!

Specifically, there are two main types of socializing that we need to do more of as moms. First, there's *normal socializing*. This is any type of interaction where you're getting together with other adults and talking about ideas, current events, places you've been, plans for the future, and things of that nature. It's a book group or a coffee with a friend you attend once per week. It's a recreational sports team you play on for a few months per year. It's getting together with some friends from work for lunch or drinks. It's meeting up with your college roommates to catch up and remember old times.

Then there's *group socialization*, which is also very good for the mind and soul. In addition to the types of standard social interactions, we believe that moms also need to be part of a mom tribe. We need a group that is specifically made up of other moms who have kids who are roughly the same ages as our own. It's important to get together regularly with your tribe in a purely social context to unload your stress and trade war stories. This is fundamental to feeling that you're not alone. It helps to break up the illusion that motherhood should look like a perfect Pinterest board.

BRING WHAT YOU'VE GOT, BY M

I knew I needed to hang out with my friends once I became a mom. The problem was that once I moved to Miami, my husband had all of his new friends at work or maybe from his passion for kite surfing, but I had little chance to get to know other moms like me. I would go to the park, beach, and pool with my babies, and maybe a kind elderly neighbor would chat a bit with me.

Years passed and I got lucky. I started making more friends and being able to share this motherhood journey daily. My friends and I would get together for a quick drink every once in a while and talk for a couple of hours. Everyone brought whatever they wanted to drink and even eat. It was like a funny adult picnic on someone's balcony. But instead of planned meals, we had a piece of already opened cheese from someone's fridge, one or two cans of Diet Coke, a couple of beers, and a half eaten can of peanuts. We didn't need more; everyone had already had dinner two hours ago with their kids. We were all moms, tired moms, desperate to just get out of the house for a little while and be with friends. The agreement was "bring whatever you can, no cooking or making an extra effort allowed." The food, the drinks, even the place didn't matter. It was just about having a nice time with friends, talking about our day as moms or wives, and even discussing dreams with uninterrupted conversations. We managed to get together at least every week or two.

One Saturday afternoon, after a whole day at the beach with my family, two friends, and their kids, I sat down on my Tommy Bahama beach chair and felt the warm sun on my face. For a split second I closed my eyes and then popped them right back open. "No, no, you have to watch the kids," I thought. And that's when it hit me: "I never relax at the beach!" I thought about my day and all the hassle to convince the kids to put on their sunscreen and their floaties, wiping their bananas clean from being dropped in the sand. It was great, but this was weekly. We have always lived in a nice condo with direct access to Florida's sandy beaches and crystal waters, but as parents, beach time is hardly a relaxing kick-back-and-enjoy-the-sun experience.

And that's when I started Friday morning beach getaways with my girlfriends. It was the same concept as before with the nighttime escape to someone's balcony: "Bring what you've got or don't bring anything at all." That's the beauty of it—just you, your bathing suit, and smile. Everybody was super busy during the week while the kids were at school, but I decided that we all deserved Friday mornings off to recharge, to be able to lie down on the sand, eyes closed, and take a breath. It was the cheapest spa we'd ever paid for. It became a tradition among my group of friends.

An active group-texting thread is an essential component of any good mom tribe. The truth is that nonparents will just never be able to understand certain things you're dealing with, and there are certain issues that dads simply don't have to face. Your mom tribe is where you can make sense of all this stuff and feel fully heard, seen, and understood without guilt or judgment.

The one thing both these types of socializing have in common is that they require time and energy. And, of course, these two resources are in very short supply for moms. In order to spread some chips to your social life, you're going to need to get a handle on some consistent, high-quality childcare to free up some time in your schedule. The expenses can really start to add up if you go out with friends and spend money on food, drinks, or admission, plus you have to pay the sitter when you get back home.

Lydia Denworth talks of the importance of a social network through the studies done with apes that measure the happy hormone oxytocin in chimpanzees. When they hang out with other apes they slightly know, their oxytocin levels are steady, but when they hang out with ones they know well and that they have a good relationship with, their levels of the happy hormone shoot up.

> *"Spending time with friends does not just make you feel psychologically happy and good—but it literally [affects how] your cardiovascular system works, and your immune system, and your sleep, and your cognitive health, your mental health, even the rate at which your cells age. How fast you biologically age is affected by how socially integrated you feel."*
>
> —*Lydia Denworth,* science journalist and author[63]

---

63 Lydia Denworth, *Friendship: The Evolution, Biology, and Extraordinary Powers of Life's Fundamental Bond* (New York: W. W. Norton & Company, 2020): 239.

The idea is to spread *some* of your chips around to your social life, not *all* of your chips. As with most things, balance is key. Don't let your role as a mom isolate you from your old friends and stop you from making new ones. In fact, you'll be a better mom if you keep your social life active.

CHAPTER 9

Finding Purpose in Work

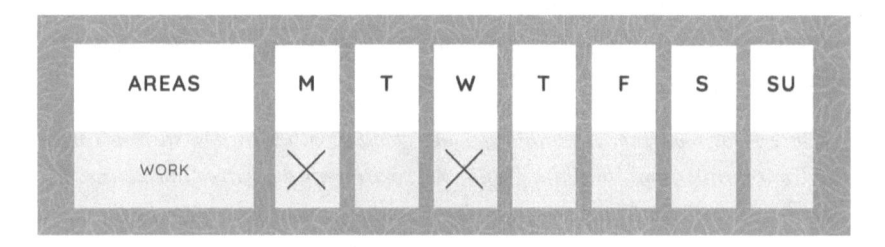

AREAS	M	T	W	T	F	S	SU
WORK	X		X				

"A happy mother is a good mother, and if work makes you hum, your whole family sings along."

—Sharon Meers and Joanna Strober, authors of Getting to 50/50

Work is an area in life where many women are able to find an additional sense of meaning, purpose, and fulfillment outside of the home. Work provides us with duties, deadlines, and the chance to be a part of something larger than ourselves. It can also mean being a member of a supportive team of people who count on you and care about you, which is another important component of life satisfaction. However, some real complexities and difficulties can arise around work-life balance.

Maybe you're already working, love your job, and can't wait to wake up every morning and rush to the office. In that case, let's look at how you can get even more enjoyment out of your profession while avoiding the risks of getting too invested in the workplace. Perhaps you work outside of the home, but you don't enjoy your job or find it fulfilling. If so, we're going to explore how to turn things around, jump to a job that fires you up, and get more joy out of what you're already doing.

But first, what if you aren't working at all right now? How can full-time moms start to spread some chips into the work category when the demands of motherhood already feel exhausting and overwhelming?

FIND YOUR VOICE, BY A SILENT Z

I had always lived abroad because my dad worked for the United Nations, and once he retired, I chose to go back home to Uruguay to get my bachelor's in communications and marketing. I had lived my entire life until then as an English speaker, and I felt it was time to get back to my roots, learn Spanish, and get to know my home country a bit more. When you study writing and communications and marketing, you're constantly bombarded by the concept of finding your voice. After a very hard introduction to the language, I discovered that I was a pretty good writer in Spanish! Who knew?

Once I got working, I found out I was good at other things, such as corporate communications, branding, and, yes, writing and creative marketing. My boyfriend at the time, now my amazing husband, was working in the financial sector, and I started to look into banks. I ended up getting a job at Santander Bank, the fifth largest bank in the world. I started at the very bottom and then grew into one of the most valued employees in the sector. I was given amazing opportunities, and I had, for the first time in my life, the feeling of being on top of the wave.

Then my husband, who was working at Wachovia at the time in Uruguay, got transferred to Wells Fargo in Miami. I had to leave my dream job, pack up, and land in a place where nobody knew my worth as a professional. I had to start from zero. It was a hard blow to my ego, going to interview after interview and not being able to make them understand the value of my career and expertise. Eventually, I got a job with LAN Airlines, a Latin American airline that had their cargo hub in Miami.

I started to thrive and show my worth until, after my firstborn, I had to decide whether to go back to the company. I continued to take small writing gigs for them. I would go to a friend's house and ask her to watch little Josefina as I sat down to work. I got another copywriting job at a small coaching company, but it was hard to manage my concentration with the baby around. I got very frustrated, and to make matters worse, I had lost my capacity to speak up for my needs and fight for myself.

My husband was in charge of our budget, and we had none to spare on childcare. The options for me to go back to work would be a simple money exchange from me to a nanny or a daycare. We had no family or friends who could help us out in a new place, and I felt stuck under the huge pressure of the babies, the house, the food, and Josefina's special needs. I lost perspective and lost my voice. Years passed and I continued to take on very small copywriting gigs. I even tried out selling on Amazon with my pal M! I realized, though, that I needed to use my time on something more moving, such as writing or inspiring or researching life's questions.

I spent a couple years soul-searching and investing in my education. During an exercise at a Tony Robbins event that my husband had gifted me for my birthday, I had a breakthrough. I wanted, needed, had to, absolutely must write a book! The funny thing is, I had always known I wanted to write a book; I had just never given it the importance it deserved. I kept looking for jobs that would give me an instant income, so I couldn't even see my husband waving from the other side saying, "Hey! It's OK! We're finally OK enough so that you can do something meaningful and not economically necessary!"

Writing a book wasn't going to tell me what to do with my life, but it was sure going to help me get back into the game, find my voice again, and get me back to me. Having a big project, a long one, in writing, was the perfect job I needed! That was December 2019. In January 2020, I ran into M, and she and I embarked on this journey together. I am at a loss for words to show how grateful I am that everything I went through these past eight years might actually help someone!

A GOOD EYE, BY M

I am the third of seven siblings. They are all very book smart, got great grades, and are top-student people, except for me. I was your regular "progressing" student who didn't stand out much at all. I'm actually grateful for this. I got used to being the one who had to hustle a bit more than the rest in my house, and this eventually made me the hustler and self-made woman I am today. Thank you to my brothers and sisters!

I studied child psychology and graduated as a child psychologist in Chile. From a practical point of view, I figured that if I helped a child live better, I would be improving almost 50 to 60 years of someone's life. If I helped an adult, on the other hand, their time to adjust and make improvements was shorter and their problems deeper.

While working in Chile, I was always told that I had a very "good eye" for the cases I had to work with. It was then that I first started seeing how many of the problems the children had were usually solvable by observing the mother and simply asking her how she felt. This usually gave me insight on the real situation and context the child was living in. Little did I know that this book was already brewing inside of my head.

We landed in Miami a short time later with an eight-month-old and a baby on the way. I was informed that in order to work as a child psychologist in the US, I had to get an entirely new degree. I knew I had more to offer than just my maternal qualities. I loved being a mom, but I needed something more as well, so I started brainstorming different ways to get back into work—ways that wouldn't require me to get another degree.

My first idea was a flop. I designed, patented, and produced a dish to serve food in for kids. I tried to get it into all the major stores, even the little ones. No one wanted my super cool dish. So much for having a good eye in retail. My first step, as I mentioned before, was my little e-book, *Picky Mimi*. Thanks to that book, I got to know the world of having a business online.

I then decided to try out this e-commerce wonder and started to make sale after sale on eBay. It was a hit. My good eye and I kept finding better and better opportunities to make an extra buck. But being a mom, I needed something that took a bit less time, and I needed to be able to control the situation on a schedule. After a bit of Googling, I learned how to sell directly from Amazon. I had products that did well and others that didn't, but everything helped to develop this new eye for online commerce that I was learning all on my own from the comfort of my own home.

Eventually my friends started to take notice. They, too, were moms who had little chance to get out of the house for work. I tutored a small group and taught them everything I knew, and they did great as well! Then one day a friend asked me if I would be willing to record everything that I had learned about selling on Amazon for an online course so that she could sell it to her sister in Boston. And that's how I fell into the world of online courses and teaching e-commerce to Spanish speakers.

Looking back at my story, what I can truly say is that I never used any of my *excuses, not the visa or the babies or the lack of help, to get me to where I am today. I always walked forward and looked around (using my good eye) to see the opportunities that were right in front of me.*

WHAT IF I DON'T WORK?

We have observed an unseen, yet very much felt, pressure for moms to be perfect at their job as sole housemakers. In an article in the *Harvard Business Review* on egalitarian couples, titled "If You Can't Find a Spouse Who Supports Your Career, Stay Single," Avivah Wittenberg-Cox shows the reader how women today, with everything at hand to be able to have a career and a family life, still tend to have trouble keeping up with their own professional path.

At one point she states, "It's not that these husbands aren't progressive, supportive spouses. They certainly see themselves that way—as do many of the CEOs and leaders of companies I work with. But they are often caught out by trade-offs they were not expecting."

According to Avivah, husbands are fine with having wives who are successful and have great salaries, and they have their backs, in theory—until it gets in the way of their own personal careers or aspirations. In her article she mentions a study by Pamela Stone and Meg Lovejoy that shows how, when it came to a woman leaving the workforce, her husband had almost 75 percent to do with the decision because "someone" had to take care of the kids. Joan Williams talks about the study, saying that even though the husbands were supportive of the career their wives had, when it came to the redistribution of chores around the house and childcare, the husbands came up short in filling in the gaps of the workload.[64]

This parenting vacuum she mentions as the load that women usually take up in the home is the dangerous obstacle that can make those of us who take on more family duties than our husbands collapse under the pressure to do it perfectly and with a smile. There's an unspoken pressure for women who want to have a career and a family life to do both tasks perfectly, and should there be an imbalance, the first option is to shame the mom into retiring her professional goals for the sake of her family. This is

---

64 Avivah Wittenberg-Cox, "If You Can't Find a Spouse Who Supports Your Career, Stay Single," *Harvard Business Review*, October 24, 2017, https://hbr.org/2017/10/if-you-cant-find-a-spouse-who-supports-your-career-stay-single.

a huge burden and a very tough choice to make. Though we applaud any conclusion that you or we may reach on this subject, we find it important to point out that the choice has to be made with a clear conscience and a fair view of what each partner can bring to the family table in terms of finding a happy medium and then take action from there. To have the sole responsibility of raising a family is huge, and we believe that no matter what the work situation is for either parent, it's a team effort, and we need to divide the load.

We're sorry if this all sounds daunting. The reality is, once you have a family, there are needs to be met and mouths to feed, so someone must keep steady income flowing into the house. We find that many factors leave us moms scrambling for our own professional calling. The real eye-opener for us in this article was the following: "Even for couples who are committed to equality, it takes two exceptional people to navigate tricky dual-career waters. It's easier to opt for the path of least resistance—the historical norm of a career-focused man and a family-focused woman. Especially if, as is often the case, the man is a few years older, has a career head start, and so earns a higher salary. This leads to a cycle that's hard to break: men get more opportunities to earn more, and it gets harder and harder for women to catch up."[65]

Today women are told, "You can do whatever you want and be whoever you want to be! You can have it all!" At the same time, the standards for doing a good job as a mom are sky high. We have all the information we could ever need to properly raise a child and be a perfect professional at the office. To make matters worse, we are pressured to measure ourselves against all the other families out there on social media. What a time to be alive!

There are many reasons why a mom might not be working right now. Maybe she has family money and doesn't need income. Or maybe her spouse has a great job and makes enough so that it doesn't make sense to pay for childcare when she can stay at home, at least for now. Maybe childcare is too expensive. Maybe she feels anxious about leaving her baby with someone she doesn't know very well. Maybe, maybe, maybe. The reasons can go on and on, but it's important to see if the reasons are actually real or if they're excuses. We want you to focus on what you do have and can do, no matter how small or short, because the path has to start somewhere.

---

65 Wittenberg-Cox, "If You Can't Find a Spouse."

Let's face it: being a mom is hard work in and of itself! As soon as you leave your job, your mom duties quickly expand to fill all of your new "free time." Soon, it's almost impossible to imagine adding a job back into your life on top of everything else. But it *is* possible, and it's extremely important to do so, both for yourself and for your family. Thankfully, our research shows that basic part-time work, community service, and volunteer work are just as beneficial as a full-time career.

Other studies have found the same thing. One 2012 Gallup survey of 60,000 women found that moms who didn't work reported significantly higher rates of depression and feelings of isolation compared to nonmothers and moms who did work. Even if a mom didn't particularly like her job or was employed only part time, she consistently reported lower levels of sadness and frustration in addition to higher levels of thriving than moms who didn't work at all. And those were just short-term benefits.[66]

In three separate longitudinal studies, two in the United States and one in the United Kingdom, researchers found that women who worked during motherhood reported being physically and mentally healthier and having higher energy levels and lower rates of depression compared to moms who did not work. These results held true for all mothers, regardless of income, education level, age, or ethnicity.[67]

The effects spill over to the children as well. One recent study reported that women whose mothers held a job during their youth demonstrate better employment outcomes as adults compared with women whose moms didn't work. The daughters of working moms were found to have higher incomes, occupy superior positions, do less housework, and have more egalitarian views than the daughters of nonworking moms. Similarly, the study found that men who grew up with a mom who worked helped out more around the house as adults and were more likely to also have a wife who worked compared to men whose mother didn't hold a job.

Importantly, moms and their children received all of these long-term and short-term benefits regardless of whether the moms were working full time

---

[66] Elizabeth Mendes et al., "Stay-At-Home Moms Report More Depression, Sadness, Anger," Gallup, May 18, 2012, https://news.gallup.com/poll/154685/stay-home-moms-report-depression-sadness-anger.aspx.

[67] Adrianne Frech and Sarah Damaske, "The Relationships between Mothers' Work Pathways and Physical and Mental Health," *Journal of Health and Social Behavior* 53, no. 4 (2012): 396–412, https://doi.org/10.1177/0022146512453929.

or part time during motherhood. Their salary didn't matter, and whether she liked her job or not didn't matter.[68] Science shows consistently that having any kind of job—even a crappy one—is better than not having any job.

More research expands on these considerations. According to a systematic review by researchers at the University of California, Irvine, toddlers and infants who have working moms do the same in terms of behavior as children who have stay-at-home moms. Taking into account 69 studies conducted over 50 years, the result on kids' school performance and behavioral problems was very balanced.[69] These studies tell us that your child will be fine whether you stay at home or go to work, so the decision is really up to you, and you can't use your child as an excuse. Focus on yourself and what you need to feel fulfilled because your child doesn't necessarily need for you to stay put at home.

Now that you know the benefits of work, you may even consider working without having to go to an actual office. The freelance economy is exploding. Millions of moms now work for themselves as entrepreneurs, bloggers, consultants, graphic artists, or virtual assistants. The landscape of the working world is changing dramatically, and no matter your situation, you can find an easy way to spread some of your chips to the work category without making it a big deal.

By work, we're talking about anything you can do in exchange for money or not. It doesn't have to be a lot of money, and it doesn't have to be a lot of time. In fact, the work doesn't even have to be something you love in order to take advantage of the numerous benefits. But work is an important space for moms to spread some chips to and find some purpose. We just want you to get your feet in the door. If you are at home with two babies thinking, "When will I ever go back to work?" you can start your process of getting back on your professional feet by taking small steps. You don't have to go out and start shooting your CV everywhere like crazy without even knowing what you want or how you can manage your mom time and work time. Take your time to carefully work out the steps you want to take. But

---

[68] Kathleen McGinn et al., "Learning from Mum: Cross-National Evidence Linking Employment and Adult Children's Outcomes," *Work Employment and Society* 33, no. 3 (April 2018): 374–400, https://doi.org/10.1177/0950017018760167.

[69] "The Kids Are All Right: Few Negative Associations With Moms' Return to Work Soon After Having Children," American Psychological Association, 2010, https://www.apa.org/news/press/releases/2010/10/working-mothers.

take the steps. Don't let overthinking stop you from doing.

Spreading some chips in this area means that even thinking about what you would be interested in doing after the baby years is helpful. We don't want to push you and stress you about going back to work because the reality is that there are different types of women who have different types of necessities and ways of functioning. We all have one friend who was back to work one month after giving birth. Similarly, most of us know a mom or two who never returned to work. The point is, we are all busy, and as moms of four, we can guarantee that your life will never get easy. You'll always have the same 24 hours, and there will always be blocks in your way, but if you keep your mind open to the idea of working on something you enjoy (even if it's not paid), your life will gain another dimension. You might get to know a part of you that had been asleep for a while, and the pure joy of getting to hang out with your own productive, badass self outside of the mom arena might be just what the doctor ordered!

Again, work is about so much more than a paycheck. Many self-made millionaires who are set for life decide to continue working long after they could have retired to a life of golf, leisure, and relaxation. Even people who win the lottery often don't completely quit their jobs. Work can provide a deep sense of purpose, a community of like-minded others, and a series of challenging goals to achieve—a great return on your chips, if you ask us.

In some ways, motherhood is like your favorite flavor of ice cream—cold, sweet, and mouth-wateringly decadent. You love it and want it. In moderation, it's easily your favorite food on the planet. But if you eat too much of it, you're in for a nasty stomachache. The next day you might notice that, weirdly enough, you crave a salad with some fresh carrots.

Work, whether you love it or tolerate it, is like that nutritious salad. It might not be your favorite thing, but you know it's good for you. After you've eaten it, you feel healthy and proud. You're taking good care of your body. Hoorah! And when you switch back to ice cream for dessert, wow, does it have a renewed appeal. You might say eating salad makes you appreciate the ice cream even more.

A study conducted by Jennifer Caputo of the Max Planck Institute for Demographic Research shows that the positive effects of work experience follow women for their whole lives. Caputo closely studied a sample of over 5,000 diverse women between the years of 1967 and 2003 from the

National Longitudinal Survey of Mature Women in the US to determine the relationship, if any, between employment history and physical and mental health. Women who had been employed for a prolonged period—regardless of income, general satisfaction with work experience, or other potentially confounding variables—lived longer and with fewer physical limitations later in life. By 2012, members of the original research group had a 25 percent lower risk of death was than women who had never worked outside the home.[70] Beyond the immediate benefits of employment, a chance for a longer and more satisfying life is certainly a reward for women who work.

For most big changes in life, the hardest part is getting started, and finding work as a mom is no different. This can be an exceptionally tough journey to begin. Today's economy is brutal. Not all areas of the world have equal opportunities—not even close. You may even have been out of the workforce for a while so that your résumé feels dated.

If getting an actual, physical, brick-and-mortar, punch-in-and-punch-out kind of job seems impossible for you right now, it's not a problem. You can get started completely online. Sites like freelancer.com, upwork.com, workingnotworking.com, peopleperhour.com, 99designs.com, and fiverr.com are all favorites for employers who need work done but aren't looking to hire a full-time employee. Participating in the digital economy is universally accessible for most anyone these days. Simply set up an account, choose an hourly rate, and start applying for projects.

If your kids aren't in school yet and finding affordable childcare is an issue, start off with things you can do from home. Don't be afraid to hire a babysitter for a few hours per day to give you time to retreat to your home office. If you're fortunate enough to have free or very cheap childcare in the form of a relative, use it! The idea is to start small. Maybe you'll start off making little to no money and you won't see the point, but trust us that every step you take will help you grow, develop, and hopefully increase your income.

Even if you have very little prior work experience, you can always pitch yourself on the sites listed previously for things like administrative assis-

---

70 Jennifer Caputo et al., "Midlife Work and Women's Long-Term Health and Mortality," *Demography* 57 (2020): 373–402, https://doi.org/10.1007/s13524-019-00839-6.

tance, customer service, text editing, writing, tutoring, graphic design, web development, virtual coaching, or social media management. There are so many skills you already have that are waiting to be used and improved!

If digital work doesn't appeal to you, why not do something with your hands? You could start a small business baking cakes and cookies and sweet breads or fixing up furniture to resell on Facebook Marketplace or Craigslist. If you've always wanted to spend more time on the sewing machine, start making one-of-a-kind baby clothes and selling them on the Internet. Whatever you like to do, just get started. Then post about it everywhere you can. Build yourself a simple website using Wix or Shopify and start sending traffic to it.

There is so much work out there and so many people who need what you can offer. Do an Internet search for how to hire someone who does what you're interested in doing. For instance, if you want to try your hand at being a virtual assistant, head over to Google and type in "how to hire a virtual assistant." Spend some time checking out the competition and seeing how other people are marketing themselves. Gather a list of the top marketplaces where people hire this type of worker and start making profiles. Books like Chris Guillebeau's *Side Hustle*,[71] Dan Fleyshman's *How to Set-Up Your Business for Under $1000*,[72] and Tim Ferriss' *The 4-Hour Work Week*[73] are also packed with ideas on stuff you can do on your own, usually from home, if going to work is not an option.

In most of the studies on the effects of working on moms and their families, the researchers have looked at the benefits of doing work outside of the house. The effects of remote freelance work are not as well understood, as the field is so new. In general, it's safe to assume that interacting face-to-face with other adults and making a long-term commitment to a single company or organization is probably the most ideal type of work situation, if you can arrange it. However, this research is still ongoing.

One of the biggest obstacles to getting back into the workforce might not be your skills, experience, or lack of opportunities. Rather, it may be you!

---

71 Chris Guillebeau, *Side Hustle: Build A Side Business And Make Extra Money Without Quitting Your Day Job* (London: Pan Macmillan, 2019).
72 Dan Fleyshman and Branden Hampton, *How To Set-Up Your Business For Under $1000* (self-published, 2016).
73 Timothy Ferriss, *The 4-Hour Workweek: Escape 9–5, Live Anywhere, and Join the New Rich* (New York: Harmony, 2009).

A WORLD OF DESIRES AND A BACKPACK FULL OF EXCUSES, BY M

Z and I were having dinner the other night with our friend Ximena Paul, a Kellogg MBA graduate, a mom of three, and CEO of Education First. Of course, Ximena and Z are friends not only because their names start with the last letters of the alphabet, but because they, like me, are women who are constantly searching, working, and—no matter what our situation is—moving forward.

In less than four years, we have seen Ximena land in Miami with a great education and job expertise in the education industry and work her way up to where she is today. Ximena had two kids under three when she moved to Miami. She got herself a babysitter for a couple of hours a day on a tight budget and went out to do volunteer work in various organizations. She networked like crazy, made every minute outside of her home count, and went to every single event on working moms, women, and education. She eventually became CEO for Education First, where she oversees all operations in daycares for the company in South Florida. She got into Kellogg's Executive MBA program and had her third child while she was at it.

Ximena told us about her take on women getting back to work. "I've had loads of people contact me wanting to know how to get back on the work wagon after motherhood. They tell me they feel bored or lost, and I sit down with them, give them all of the info I can think of, sometimes for over an hour every couple of days. I do it gladly because I figure I would have wanted or needed the same thing. There are lots of women that have been out of the job market for so long that they haven't really learned the ropes for the opportunities now listed for them on LinkedIn, for example. And I get it, once you get out of the job market it might be intimidating to go back in. But I'm telling you guys, there's something else that's going on because I have given a million ideas and tips and contacts to numerous moms, and they eventually either never contact me ever again, and I see that they haven't gotten into anything, or they tell me that they simply can't find the time to do anything. Most of the time I get responses like "I simply don't have time; motherhood is simply too much right now."

What I've seen is that when women know exactly what they are looking for, they get it. The problem is that most of the time, women don't know exactly what they want, especially when it comes to work. If we could focus and determine what we want, we'll use all of our resources to get it."

This got us into a huge conversation about the reasons moms sometimes fail to get back to work, volunteer, or participate in anything outside of their house. We wondered how much of the feeling of being stuck has to do with solvable excuses and how much has to do with the identity shift from matrescence.

Just remember, no one should place too many chips in any one area. Take an honest look at your career and make sure it isn't overshadowing the other areas of your life. Keeping your chips spread around helps buffer you so that if a problem ever arises at work, or if you go through a challenging or unproductive period, it won't be a huge blow to your identity.

Finally, some working moms feel guilty about missing their children's firsts while stuck at the office. *What if your baby's first words or steps happen and you aren't around to witness them?* After speaking with hundreds of working and nonworking moms all around the world, we've found that a child's real first anything doesn't happen until Mommy is around to see it. That's how much of a rock star you are in your baby's eyes. Enjoy every milestone the second you see one because a baby or kid just needs your "Wow!" and "Hurray!" to sleep tight at night, and if any milestone came before, although welcome, it wasn't as magical as yours.

Hopefully as your kids grow older, they will see your drive for whatever you do, and it will inspire them to develop this level of enthusiasm for their own work and passions.

> *"It's not wrong to be passionate about your career. When you love what you do, you bring that stimulation back to your family."*
>
> —*Allison Pearson,* writer[74]

---

74 Arianna Davis, "5 Things Author Allison Pearson Knows For Sure," *O, The Oprah Magazine,* accessed October 13, 2020, http://www.oprah.com/spirit/allison-pearson-interview-author-allison-pearson.

CHAPTER 10

Your Personal Health Coach for Free

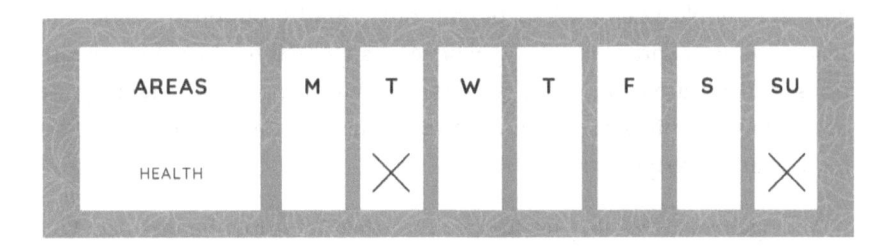

AREAS	M	T	W	T	F	S	SU
HEALTH		X					X

"Exercise gives you endorphins. Endorphins make you happy. Happy people just don't shoot their husbands."

—Elle Woods, Legally Blonde

As moms, we sometimes ignore our own health. We spend so much energy worrying about everyone else that we don't have the capacity to make our own health a priority, too. Something's gotta give, and too often we make the sacrifice. In the back of our head we know health is important, but with our busy family life and career, we may not make the time to worry about it until it's too late. Health is one of the most neglected areas.

In our study of over 600 women from around the world that we conducted in April 2020 that we mentioned in Chapter 6, 45.5 percent of respondents reported they didn't do any kind of exercise during the week. However, 82 percent of them did try to eat healthy food on a weekly basis. We were shocked to see such a high percentage of the women in our study admit they did not work out at all! On the plus side, we were relieved to see a very high percentage trying to get some healthy food into their regular meals. This could mean simply eating a salad once per week. And you know what? We'll take it because you have to start somewhere.

Broccoli does not have commercial value like pizza or frozen lasagna. We know this, so we try to keep our fridges as healthy and real as possible. The days of overly processed foods are fading away and the general public is more conscious of the healthy options available. Even fast-food restaurants try to appeal to the more aware public with salads, wraps, and meatless burgers. When you want to choose something healthy to eat these days, the sheer number of options available can be overwhelming.

The deck is stacked against us as moms because we just don't have time for any extra work. One simple thing we both started doing in our own homes a couple years back is buying only healthy options of food and snacks for our pantries. That way whenever anyone is hungry, the only options available are fruits, veggies, nuts, etc., but not a Dorito. Taking care of the entire family's meal plan, especially snacks, can be a real kick start for a healthy lifestyle.

And again, start small. Get the popcorn that doesn't come in a bag with three liters of melted butter on it. Get the one with no butter, add your own butter at home in a less generous amount, and see how that flies. Trade in a few good products for better ones. The important thing here is being aware of what we are doing to our bodies and what we are feeding ourselves.

LET'S GET PHYSICAL, BY M

Three years after my fourth baby was born, I made up my mind to commit to a regular workout routine. I know myself well enough to know that I was not going to get through it unless I had someone kicking my butt and urging me to go. I hired a personal trainer, the least expensive one around (because either you do the workout because the trainer is good at motivating you, or you do it because you see your dollars slip away with every minute), and everything went great—at first. The workouts were brutal (just picture me barely walking, mummy style, after each session). Sure, I was getting healthier, but the pain was killing me.

One day I asked him what people do to stay consistent with this training because I surely hated it and was coming up with all kinds of excuses not to con-

tinue the torture. And he told me, "Exercise is like everything in life; the more you do it, the easier it gets. But the real trick is being conscious of what you eat combined with working out." OK, great! *I thought to myself. So, I added one more day of training per week (great marketing this guy had); and eventually the workouts did get easier, and my body started to get used to it.*

But the thing that really changed my opinion on exercise and working out was being conscious about everything I ate and all the activity I did. It might seem pretty obvious, but it sure wasn't for me. When I started working out, the first thing my trainer taught me was to be fully aware of everything that went into my mouth each day. He didn't tell me to cut out anything, just to be aware. He showed me how to keep a food diary, for example. Doing a daily run-through of what I ate got me into the habit of thinking before munching, and I did see quick results!

I had never paid attention to what I put into my mouth before, and I was a bit shocked. I hadn't realized all of the snacks and crap I was eating. I was eating healthy meals, sure, but in between meals I was killing myself with bites of whatever I found—or the kids' leftovers.

EATING AND SLEEPING

Mindful.org has a list written by Christopher Willard, PsyD, that shows examples of what mindful eating looks like versus mindless eating.[75] Don't get too bummed out if you see yourself represented in the wrong column because you've been eating without even noticing just to get through the day or get things done. We've all been there, either years ago or maybe two hours ago while writing this book.

Mindless Eating	Mindful Eating
Eating past full and ignoring your body's signals	Listening to your body and stopping when full
Eating when emotions tell us to eat (i.e., sad, bored, lonely)	Eating when our bodies tell us to eat (i.e., stomach growling, energy low)
Eating alone, at random times and places	Eating with others, at set times and places

---

75 Christopher Willard, "6 Ways to Practice Mindful Eating," Mindful.org, January 17, 2019, https://www.mindful.org/6-ways-practice-mindful-eating/.

Eating foods that are emotionally comforting	Eating foods that are nutritionally healthy
Eating and multitasking	When eating, just eating
Considering a meal an end product	Considering where food comes from

It's interesting how we can worry so much about our kids' food intake, their nutritional needs, their feet off of the table and mouths closed while they chew, and at the same time have a complete absence of mind about our own meals. How many times have we felt anxiety for something and gobbled down that last ice cream bar in the fridge? How many times do we either skip meals to get everything we need to get done before the kids get out of daycare or school, and then just have whatever they're having for an afternoon snack and consider ourselves fed? How many times do we walk into the supermarket starved and open the bag of Oreos while we finish checking off the shopping list? How many times do we eat and look at our cell phones, feed babies, or get work done from the office with a salad on our laps? When we feed our kids, we measure how much they eat so they'll have enough energy to go to the park, and we check to see that the plate has a bit of protein, veggies, and fruits so that their little minds will grow as healthy as possible.

But who's taking care of our energy levels at the office, supermarket, PTA meeting, and house? Our minds may have grown all they can in size, but they still need good nutrition to thrive—so do our bodies, so does our mood. Eating healthy is like fuel for the car, and many times we're almost surprised that we can drive more miles. We have to be our own nutritionist, and it's either in the weekly meal prep and shopping list or the healthy, handy snack availability that we can get somewhere with this.

Sleep and rest are critical, too. Being a mom doesn't really allow you to get as much sleep as you want, so be aggressive about getting to sleep early, turning off the TV at a set time, and counting your hours. Know your body and respect the amount of downtime it needs. If you don't know where to start, go back to the eating healthy example. If we're so on top of our kids' sleep training and nighttime tuck-in hours, it's not because we're annoying—it's because we know they need their good rest. Nobody likes a cranky toddler on their hands because of poor sleep. The solution is easy, and we'll apply it to them on the spot. But when it comes to us, we stall in taking action on our own sleeping routines. Yes, we are grown up, but we also need to respect our body and its needs, and having a steady bedtime hour can work wonders.

While we're at it, scientists have proven that to have a good night's sleep, we need to disconnect from our screens one hour before bedtime.[76] So, turn that off and take advantage of the one-hour adult time to connect with your partner. It's basically a two-for-one combo of success. You're welcome.

YOU'VE GOT TO MOVE IT, MOVE IT

Now that we've jogged around the subjects of eating and sleeping, let's get back to the real pickle that popped up in our study: the lack of exercise. Why is this so troubling? It's because sneaking a salad here and there, skipping the chocolate cake at the party, or having a couple of bad nights' rest and then catching up with a nap on the weekend is less complicated than not working out at all for years on end. The body and the mind need exercise. Period.

How was it that 45.5 percent of the women in our study reported that they didn't do *any* sort of exercise in their entire week? Was it a lack of motivation? Was it that they didn't really understand the true value of exercise? Or was it just a bad habit of not prioritizing it?

According to Laura Vanderkam, mom of four kids and author of three books on time management, "What people mean when they say they don't have time to exercise is that they do not currently consider it a priority during their waking, nonworking hours. There may be good reasons for this; for instance, some parents worry that exercise will take time from their kids (though few people spend 50 hours per week interacting with their kids either)."[77]

Health is one of the five main areas you can spread some chips to. Most moms we've worked with find that parking at least a few chips here on the physical health category adds to their lives in a positive way. So, we want to talk about how to do it in the most efficient and effective manner possible.

---

[76] "Why screen time can disrupt sleep," Science Daily, November 27, 2018, https://www.sciencedaily.com/releases/2018/11/181127111044.htm.
[77] Laura Vanderkam, "Finding time to exercise," Laura Vanderkam, August 14, 2009, https://lauravanderkam.com/2009/08/finding-time-to-exercise/.

As mentioned in a Harvard Health Publication,[78] "regular aerobic exercise will bring remarkable changes to your body, your metabolism, your heart, and your spirits. It has a unique capacity to exhilarate and relax, to provide stimulation and calm, to counter depression and dissipate stress." Exercise increases endorphins, reduces the levels of stress hormones in our bodies, and has a positive effect on our moods. In fact, the mood-enhancing benefits of a 20-minute exercise session can last for 12 hours![79] Exercise has a powerful effect on our mental states when we are in a bad mood.

> *"An early morning walk is a blessing for the whole day"*
> —*Henry David Thoreau*

So how much exercise is enough? People who exercise for about 30 minutes five days a week get great benefits, according to the CDC.[80] But less may help you feel good, too. Research shows that even a short stroll can improve mood—so you don't have to be a personal trainer yourself. Don't aim too high; just start somewhere and get moving. And you don't do have to do it alone. Call up your friends to go for a walk together, start a carpool with the people who go to your gym, and try to find peers to enjoy the process with.

With the Internet, easy and quick home workouts are just a few keystrokes away. There are exercises to do with dumbbells as well as exercises to do with a baby, a heavy book, or your own body weight. If doing exercise on your own seems too boring, find a buddy or work out with your kids. Make it a competition.

If you know that you'd rather exercise as part of a group or in an organized sport, find a class or join a league. Public recreation centers, studios, and gyms all have these options, and they are affordable and easy to sign up for. Facebook is also a good place to find groups of people in your town

---

78 Avivah Wittenberg-Cox, "If You Can't Find a Spouse Who Supports Your Career, Stay Single," *Harvard Business Review*, October 24, 2017, https://hbr.org/2017/10/if-you-cant-find-a-spouse-who-supports-your-career-stay-single.

79 Jeremy S. Sibold and Kathleen M. Berg, "Mood Enhancement Persists for up to 12 Hours Following Aerobic Exercise: A Pilot Study," Perceptual and Motor Skills 111, no. 2 (October 2010): 333–42, https://doi.org/10.2466/02.06.13.15.pms.111.5.333-342.

80 "How Much Physical Activity Do Adults Need?" Centers for Disease Control and Prevention, October 7, 2020, https://www.cdc.gov/physicalactivity/basics/adults/index.htm.

who want to play volleyball or kickball but don't necessarily want to play in a paid league.

For others, it can really be helpful to work with a personal trainer or join a small group exercise class. Again, check out what your local fitness center offers for free or minimal charge. Call up a yoga studio and see if they have any free classes on public spaces. Take your kid with you.

> *"Exercise because you appreciate your body, not because you judge it."*
>
> —Unknown

But first, get more conscious about the exercise you're already doing. For example, picking up a 20-pound child is actually more difficult than lifting a 20-pound dumbbell—the dumbbell doesn't try to squirm out of your arms. Every day you pick up things like car seats, bags of groceries, and toys. You make beds, push strollers, mop floors, and wipe countertops. Believe it or not, these are legitimate forms of exercise. And thinking of them as exercise can help you get more benefits from them.

In an ingenious experiment with 84 female hotel maids, Harvard psychologist Ellen Langer showed how a simple shift in mindset can make a big difference in the effects of our actions.[81] When asked if they got any exercise, most of the maids initially said no. But then Langer gave 44 of them a lesson about how the work they already did every day—pushing around vacuums, scrubbing tubs and sinks, making beds, moving furniture, etc.—counted as exercise and had big benefits for their health. The maids even sat down with a researcher who explained to them exactly how many calories each of these routine tasks burned. The other 40 maids were given no information or messages on the fact that their jobs included a lot of exercise.

When researchers followed up with the maids a few weeks later, the 44 women who had been told to think of their work as exercise demonstrated significantly lower blood pressure, lower weight, and lower stress than they had at the start of the experiment. The control group had no such effects. Further, a follow-up revealed that the exercising maids didn't significantly

---

[81] Alix Spiegel, "Hotel Maids Challenge the Placebo Effect," NPR, January 3, 2008, https://www.npr.org/templates/story/story.php?storyId=17792517.

increase their activity level after learning these facts. They simply changed the way they thought about their own behavior.

The same is true for you. You are already exercising a lot. It's not helpful to think of yourself as someone who doesn't do any activity because then you are subconsciously telling yourself that you have a very long way to go before you reach fitness. It's much better to realize that you're not starting from zero. Notice where you already get exercise. There's surely plenty of activity in your daily life. Give yourself credit for all of that hard work.

Now just add a few full-on dedicated workout sessions into the mix each week and you'll be on fire! Recognizing that you already do plenty of exercise in your daily routine can open up your eyes to how easy it is to slip in a bit more—and maybe even make carrying those heavy groceries a bit more rewarding. Being halfway there is motivating, isn't it?! This phenomenon is known as the endowed progress effect, and it has been studied extensively.

It's also true that, for many moms, investing a little bit more of yourself on eating right and exercise can give you a nice sense of fulfillment and joy. We believe women should love themselves no matter what. We should be the first to give each other a bit of slack and understand that beauty comes in all shapes and sizes. We also know that working out on a regular schedule, be it once, twice, or three times a week, can have a huge impact on our overall health, longevity, flexibility, mobility, and mood. Ladies, our mood! We need all the positive players we can get in the mood department! Motherhood asks us to keep our cool when our patience and energy are pushed to their last limits. Working out can really give us a place to decompress and let go of all the thoughts we process each day.

Your current body is a result of your current habits. Often, our habits were passed on to us by our parents.[82] By our mid-20s, many of us are firmly set in our food habits, so whatever your parents' habits were before they had kids, that is likely the food legacy that was passed on to you. And whatever your habits were before you had kids, those are probably the habits that you will pass along to your own children.

It can be very difficult to break routines, and this is especially true when it comes to food. Changing up your diet and exercise routine is a disrup-

---

[82] Jennifer S. Savage, et al., "Parental Influence on Eating Behavior," *The Journal of Law, Medicine & Ethics* 35, no. 1 (2007): 22–34, https://doi.org/10.1111/j.1748-720X.2007.00111.x.

tion to your usual way of life. This makes any changes inherently difficult to start and maintain. Did you know that almost 80 percent of people who join a gym will quit within five months? This disruption is also why people who join a gym more than four miles away from their home tend to work out significantly less often compared with those who have a membership at a gym that's two and one-half miles away or less. If the gym is conveniently located, you can stop in on your way to work or bundle a quick workout with some other errands. If the gym is out of the way, you'll have to plan a special trip.

Of course, if there's not a gym close by it doesn't mean you're doomed to be inactive. It just means you might have to get more creative. In the wake of coronavirus, people everywhere have discovered the benefit of at-home workouts on YouTube.

SHELTER IN PLACE, BY Z

After my fourth baby, I was exhausted. Life had finally run me down, and I couldn't get back to working out, even though I knew it would lift my energy level and make me feel much better. But for some reason I simply couldn't get myself to move. I just didn't have it in me. I needed a break from everything.

When my fourth turned one and a half, I found a cute little playgroup to drop the kids at from 9 a.m. to 12:30 p.m. I couldn't believe it; I finally had three full hours a day for myself! I started to work on new projects such as this book, catch up with old friends over coffee, take care of doctor's appointments, make supermarket and pharmacy runs, and anything else I needed. Working out was definitely on the top of my list, and I wanted to do it every day. But I quickly realized that taking an entire hour for a workout would leave me with barely two for the rest of my huge to-do list.

I eventually started to prioritize work and errands. I also needed to feel that I had my life back, and getting things crossed off my to-do list gave me a very addictive feeling of satisfaction. And this is when my workout sessions started to slowly disappear from my schedule again. "It's not my fault! I have too little time for myself!" I said, making excuses for myself.

Then one day, everything changed. My schedule, the kids' schedule, our entire lives were put on hold by the COVID-19 pandemic. The minutes in my day were suddenly 100 percent dedicated to my four little people in my three-bedroom apartment. They began remote learning, and I became a teacher over-

night. *Everything I had been working on was put on hold. But something inside of me knew this was no time to mess around with my body, mental health, and personal care. Funny how I needed a global crisis to get back into my sneakers. Some people just work better under pressure, I guess.*

I found some amazing workout videos during my kids' TV time and consistently completed at least 20 minutes of working out every day. I even started to get back to work on my projects (such as this book). These days, my workout time is sacred. I know that if I don't take that time for myself, my Rubik's Cube is going to get jumbled up.

CHANGING THE HABIT

Many women also have some feelings when it comes to food, exercise, and the entire idea of fitness. We can blame Barbie, the media, and celebrities for making us all feel self-conscious about our bodies. Maybe your mom, sister, friends, or family tends to talk a bit too much about the subject as well. But wherever these feelings come from, they are real and very influential on our behavior.

Starting to behave in healthier ways is really hard. Friends might judge you, your kids (and partner) might complain, and you might have a hard time tuning in to what foods are working for you because your taste buds will rebel at first. Keep at it. It takes the better part of a week to notice the changes of doing a full 180 in your diet. Small changes will take longer to notice, and it takes at least 30 days for any new behavior to become a habit. Luckily, there is a reward in eating healthy for health's sake. It's like every time you eat that salad, you get a little gold star from yourself. You did it, and your body is better for it.

Movement is the name of the game. Some exercises are better than others, but any exercise is always better than no exercise. So, get mindful about moving and see how much you can work into your existing routine. Carve out time to exercise your favorite way—if not for you, just do it for the kids.

> *"One of the best reasons to exercise is that it models healthy behaviors for your children—you don't want them to grow up and think that it's optional!"*
> —Laura Vanderkam[83]

---

83 Vanderkam, "Finding time to exercise."

THE FAMOUS WHY

Exercising is often equated with slimming down in our culture. If a woman tells you she just joined a gym or started working out, you'll probably assume she's trying to lose weight. You might say something like, "Girl, why? You look fabulous!" or "You of all people definitely do *not* need to work out." In other words, we automatically focus on how exercise affects appearance.

But the real payback for working out is overall health, including on the inside. It keeps your entire body in tip-top shape. It affects your mood, your stress management, and your coordination. Another reason to work out are those icky statistics that nobody really wants to talk about, such as how strenuous workouts like weightlifting are hugely important especially for women, who are prone to osteoporosis later in life. Just get moving whenever and however you can.

Depending on where you come from and your family traditions, you might sometimes feel that certain people don't exactly have your back once you start your shift toward a workout routine of some sort. It may even seem like others sometimes try to convince you not to work out. Comments such as "You don't need to work out! You're perfect," can be heard from Aunt Ednas all over the world. Are they trying to make us feel better? Most of the time they are actually trying to make *themselves* feel better. They usually have their own issues surrounding exercise and diet, and it's not really about you. They may feel guilty about not showing as much commitment as you are or not being in the kind of shape they want to be in. If they can convince you to stay the same, then they won't have to confront their own habits and face the hard reality of their own life. Misery really does love company.

A wise person once said that we are the sum total of the five people we surround ourselves with. If your spouse, your best friends, your kids, and your coworkers are all unhealthy, it's going to feel like you're fighting against the current when you start making positive changes in your own life. There's no easy answer for how to handle this. Maybe you have to exercise without telling these people, or maybe you can join an online health community like Weight Watchers and find encouragement there. Whatever you do, don't do this alone. Call up the friends who you know will be supportive, talk to the people at your gym, and try to find peers to enjoy the process with.

ENDOWED PROGRESS

In one study, researchers handed out punch cards to customers at a car wash and measured how many people completed the punch cards and cashed them in.[84] The punch cards were like the ones used by many cafés. Once a customer filled it up with enough punches, they received a free car wash. However, there were two different versions of the punch card. On the first one, customers needed eight punches to get a free car wash. On the second, they needed 10 punches, but the card came with the first two pre-punched. In other words, the second group got the feeling of a small head start, even though both actually needed the same number of car washes before they would receive a free one.

The results of the study showed that the customers who were randomly given the second type of card—with two free punches—were a full 82 percent more likely to finish the card and redeem it for a free car wash. That's a *huge* effect. By making them feel like they weren't starting completely from zero, the researchers helped them stay motivated to fill up their cards.

Physical health is an area of life we may not pay attention to until something goes wrong. Historically, humans lived such short life spans that we didn't have to worry about keeping our bodies healthy through our 50s, 60s, and 70s. But the world has changed. We are living a lot longer, and we have to be proactive in order to keep ourselves healthy for as long as possible.

We can save our future selves a lot of heartache (and joint pain) by investing some chips on our physical health today.

---

84 Joseph C. Nunes and Xavier Drèze, "The Endowed Progress Effect: How Artificial Advancement Increases Effort," *Journal of Consumer Research* 32 (March 2006).

CHAPTER 11

Mental Wellness
Is a Priority

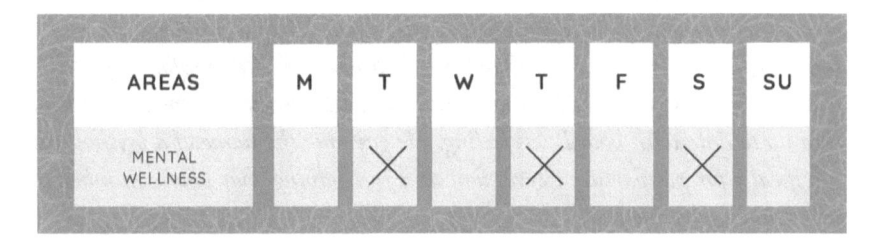

AREAS	M	T	W	T	F	S	SU
MENTAL WELLNESS		X		X		X	

Motherhood usually comes with two bonus packages called anxiety and depression. Worldwide, about 10 percent of pregnant women and 13 percent of women who have just given birth experience a mental disorder, primarily depression.[85] First off, you're sleeping much less than you've slept for almost 99 percent of your life before kids. You are responsible for this little person, and if anything goes wrong, the feeling is that it's all on you. All of this anxiety placed in a blender, plus a little bit of a chemical imbalance provoked by your postpartum hormones, can be a recipe for depression.

Let's jump forward to a couple of years after you've had kids. At this point you've been taking care of those little rascals nonstop for days on end. Their goals are your goals, and their life is your life. As a mom, you will move agendas around to find your kid an appointment with their doctor when they start showing signs that something is amiss. But can you honestly say you would rush to do the same for yourself? We are moms,

---
[85] "Maternal and child mental health," World Health Organization, accessed October 13, 2020, https://www.who.int/mental_health/maternal-child/en/.

not superheroes. Sometimes we need to pay attention to our own needs.

Your mental health needs your chips. In many ways this is your most important category of all. When talking about your identity, mental health is a crucial piece of the puzzle. No matter how many chips you invest in being present with your kids, connecting with your partner, working out, eating your spinach, meditating, and going out with friends, if your mental health is off, none of the other categories will click into flow mode.

BE YOUR OWN SHRINK, BY M

Because I had studied child psychology, you could say that I was lucky in the sense that I knew pretty well the dangers of falling into a mental health issue. When my fourth child was born, I felt that I had reached a level of tiredness that I had not experienced with the first three, and if not taken care of with enough seriousness, it could have eventually turned into a problem. He had a heavy reflux issue, and this affected his sleep and my sleep profoundly. But I was quick to ask for help. No questions asked, I talked to my doctor and kept him up to date with how I was feeling. He gave me the name of a psychologist specifically for postpartum depression, and just having that phone number in my contacts gave me relief.

Another thing that I did was keep myself busy, even in my most tired moments, with something that would interest me, be it Googling something online or planning something ahead for the days when my sleep patterns would normalize. Having my older kids running around was a promise that there would come better days when I would not feel like this. I kept repeating to myself, "Remember, this is just temporary." And so it was.

You can take care of your mental health in many ways. We are going to talk about our favorites and the ones that have really worked out for us as moms.

TAKE A SOCIAL MEDIA AND SCREEN BREAK

The twin topics of anxiety and depression have been making waves in the media in recent years as the pace of life continues to quicken. Diagnoses for learning difficulties and personality disorders have been on the rise,[86,][87] and many experts blame social media for the current mental illness pandemic.[88] But the truth is we don't really know what is causing this. It seems to be a symptom of modern life.

You've probably heard about the dangers of screen addiction. Maybe your sister-in-law gave up social media for Lent. You may have noticed parenting experts talking about radical digital downtime and screen-free Sundays. We were skeptical of all the hype at first, but after exploring the research more deeply and trying some screen breaks ourselves, we realized there is a good reason people are talking about forcing themselves to take space away from social media.

Social media use has been linked to increased dissatisfaction with life.[89] Because people tend to post only the major highlights of their lives on social media, our profiles have become a highly curated body of work, which makes the real world automatically feel inferior by comparison. People don't post pictures of when they look ugly or feel down. Even those celebrities posting pictures of themselves with no makeup do so with amazing lighting, great angles, and—let's face it—excellent cheekbones.

We know that social media is only showing us a perfectly packaged final product. We are well aware that most people are working really hard behind the scenes to deliver that product. But the studies show that knowing these things isn't enough to inoculate us to social media's devastating effects. The more we are exposed to a scrolling feed, the more likely we are to suffer from stress, anxiety, and feelings of unworthiness.

Listen, we don't live in some fantasy dream world where we believe

---

86 "What's Behind the Stark Rise in Children's Disabilities," NPR, August 19, 2014, https://www.npr.org/2014/08/19/341674577/whats-behind-the-stark-rise-in-childrens-disabilities.

87 Sebastian Montes, "Facing a rising tide of personality disorders," *Counseling Today*, November 1, 2013, https://ct.counseling.org/2013/11/facing-a-rising-tide-of-personality-disorders/.

88 E. J. Mundell, "More Evidence Links Social Media Use to Poorer Mental Health in Teens," U.S. News, February 10, 2020, https://www.usnews.com/news/health-news/articles/2020-02-10/more-evidence-links-social-media-use-to-poorer-mental-health-in-teens.

89 Sabrina Barr, "Six Ways Social Media Negatively Affects Your Mental Health," *The Independent*, October 8, 2020, https://www.independent.co.uk/life-style/health-and-families/social-media-mental-health-negative-effects-depression-anxiety-addiction-memory-a8307196.html.

everyone on earth should just delete their social media accounts, cancel their Netflix subscriptions, and sit around the campfire every night telling stories and singing "Kumbaya." We get it; social media is here to stay, and we *all* need a little Netflix sometimes. But the good news is that there is mounting evidence that taking time off from screens can significantly increase your satisfaction with life.

Just being aware of the amount of time you spend looking at your phone is a great start. That might inspire you to start shutting it off for a few hours at a time or at a certain time every night so you can shift to reading books and playing with the kids. You might want to use the settings that come built into most phones now to limit certain apps to be available only during certain times of the day. These are small steps, but the data is showing they really matter.

A study from IDC Research sponsored by Facebook stated that 80 percent of smartphone users check their mobile devices within 15 minutes of waking up each morning[90]—and that's a big problem. According to Dr. Nikole Benders-Hadi, "[I]mmediately turning to your phone when you wake up can start your day off in a way that is more likely to increase stress and leave you feeling overwhelmed."[91]

So, if you want to avoid starting your day feeling anxious, rushed, or stressed, stop checking your smartphone right after waking up. Instead, go meditate, work out, wake up the kids, prepare breakfast, get showered and dressed, and then, eventually, when you really have to kick-start your day, look at your phone. Just a suggestion!

SPREAD KINDNESS

A variety of studies show that being altruistic makes us happier. When we find small ways to serve others without asking for anything in return, we'll start to reap the benefits. In one study, people were given 20 dollars and instructed to either spend the money on themselves or to spend it

---

[90] "Always Connected: How Smartphones and Social Keep Us Engaged," IDC Research Report, accessed October 13, 2020, https://www.nu.nl/files/IDC-Facebook%20 Always%20Connected%20(1).pdf.

[91] Annakeara Stinson, "Is It Bad To Look At Your Phone When You Wake Up? It Might Be Sabotaging Your Day," Elite Daily, March 8, 2018, https://www.elitedaily.com/p/is-it-bad-to-look-at-your-phone-right-when-you-wake-up-it-might-be-sabotaging-your-day-8437383.

on someone else. The people who had used the money for someone else reported feeling better about themselves and were in a more positive mood the following day than those who had invested the cash directly into their own happiness.[92] This shows that doing something nice and unexpected for another person can have a big effect on our own mental well-being.

Most kind acts don't even cost 20 dollars to pull off. You can hold the door open for someone or ask the cashier at the supermarket how her day is going—like *really* going. Or help an elderly person grab something from the back of the shelf at the grocery store. It takes only a second to be kind, and we promise you'll feel all fuzzy inside.

Spreading a little kindness can also have a positive impact on your physical health. In *TIME* magazine's robust "Guide to Happiness" from 2019, one study showed that doing multiple small acts of kindness daily helps lower blood pressure and reduce stress.[93]

NAME THAT FEELING

We've noticed a big benefit from consciously working on our emotional awareness. Try checking in with yourself a few times throughout the day. Are you angry? Sad? Excited? Anxious? Scared? Then ask yourself what triggered you to be in such an emotional state. Is it the mess in a room? Your child crying? Did you get a comment from your partner you didn't expect? Take a second to practice these two steps, and you will start to understand what's going on with you and how you can get to a better place emotionally.

This practice isn't easy, and it takes a long time to master. But keeping at it can help you achieve a more mindful and compassionate approach to dealing with your feelings. If you can fully recognize and be at peace with everything you're feeling, you'll be one step closer to truly understanding yourself.

---

92 Colleen Walsh, "Money Spent on Others Can Buy Happiness," Harvard Gazette, April 17, 2008, https://news.harvard.edu/gazette/story/2008/04/money-spent-on-others-can-buy-happiness/#:~:text=%E2%80%9CWe%20found%20that%20people%20who,it%20that%20made%20them%20happier.%E2%80%9D

93 Jenny Santi, "The Secret to Happiness Is Helping Others," *TIME*, accessed December 8, 2020, https://time.com/collection/guide-to-happiness/4070299/secret-to-happiness/

GRATITUDE

From a psychological standpoint, it's no secret that being grateful is strongly and consistently associated with greater happiness. Gratitude helps us feel more positive emotions, improve our health, deal with adversity, and build strong relationships.

The Harvard Medical School suggests some ways to cultivate gratitude on a regular basis.

1. **Write a thank-you note.** Try it! It'll make you feel good to write down what you appreciate or are thankful for from another person. It can show you what good things they have that you can therefore enjoy.

2. **Thank someone mentally.** Just take a second to close your eyes and act out in your head a nice moment to thank someone in your life.

3. **Keep a gratitude journal.** Discover the art of writing it down. The daily practice of writing what you're grateful for helps you keep all the good things in your life fresh in your mind. Handwriting processes everything in a totally different light, so don't knock it until you've tried it!

4. **Count your blessings.** Again, just write down or number in your head all the good things that you have going on. We're so fast to think about what's missing, so look at the good blessings in your life as a weekly habit instead.

5. **Meditate.** Sit down in silence and concentrate on your breathing because it gives you the immediate gratification of being able to control something absolutely controllable.

6. **Pray.** Sit, kneel, or just be still and talk out loud, asking for, thanking for, and just contemplating everything around you with love and peace.[94]

---

[94] "Giving thanks can make you happier," Harvard Health Publishing, accessed October 13, 2020, https://www.health.harvard.edu/healthbeat/giving-thanks-can-make-you-happier.

TWO IS A BUNDLE, BY Z

I had two types of pregnancy experiences. The first two were mostly rolling with the punches, surviving, and learning the ropes. The second two were very close together—they're a year and two weeks apart—but this second chapter in my pregnancies and family management caught me being much stronger and aware of what was coming. I had always wanted four children, and though the little red line on the pee stick had come up almost 12 months earlier than expected with my fourth, I had faith that I had already mastered having two babies close together with the first two. Though the first six to 12 months of my fourth child's life would be challenging, the outcome would be great. I love having my two little sets three years apart.

What I also saw coming was that, knowing my pregnancies were very hard to walk through because of my hyperemesis gravidarum (see also Chapter 3), I had to take extra care of myself. And this time was even more difficult. I had three kids who needed me and depended on me, and for their sake, I was not going to crumble.

My last pregnancy took a lot of hard work. My husband was on the first year of his MBA, working every day at the office and travelling a lot for work or to study. The nanny who had helped us until then was not able to continue working with us, the kids were small, and I was basically on my own the last trimester and constantly putting out fires. When my fourth was born, I suffered from mastitis for the first time and could not believe the amount of pain I was going through. I felt I could not be there for the rest of my kids because I had to take care of my boobies and the newborn, and I started to feel extra low in energy and emotionally.

My doctor explained to me that sometimes mastitis occurs with moms who are extremely tired and don't unload the extra milk from their breasts after a feeding. This is exactly what happened with me. For the first time in my four births, I went to sleep one night after feeding the baby, knowing that he had left milk in my boobs, but I was way too tired to pump. The next day I woke up to the horror of a swollen red breast and tears falling down my cheeks as I fed him. We needed help big-time with the rest of the kids, so thankfully I was able to ask a couple of cousins to come live with us. This changed the whole scenario.

But it was not until maybe three months after the birth that I started to pick up on a certain sense of my own angst, unwelcome and unprovoked, from morning until the kids got back from school. It caught my attention because it was so perfectly recurrent, starting and stopping at the same time every day. I, too, lost no time in calling up a therapist who had helped me in the past, almost 10 years before, and sharing my personal observations on what I was feeling.

She heard me out and explained to me that we have a certain chemical in our brain called serotonin that is produced naturally and keeps us happy. "The thing is," she said, "I see that by what you're telling me, you've used up all of your serotonin during the last months and now your body is showing you that there's a deficit." Then I asked if it was postpartum depression, knowing that she already had my family history with depression. "Why is this showing up now and not three or four months ago when the baby was born? And what I find alarming is that I've never been so happy in my life to see that I have my four babies with me! How can I feel so sad when I consciously know that this is amazing?" She took a second and calmly answered, "It doesn't seem like postpartum depression to me right now. I wouldn't worry about putting a title on it. But what is clear is that a couple of months of taking serotonin, which is found in certain antidepressants, will basically get you out of the woods of falling into something more serious. So, let's just start off there." I took three months of serotonin for the first time in my reproductive years, and it effectively pushed me out of the water.

I find it especially important to not be scared to reach out and try available options. As long as it's to get you to a better place, there's no room for ego. As mothers, we need to be OK mentally because the first ones to pay the price are our kids. We are human and superheroes at the same time, and if you need to pop a pill at some point to keep the cape flying, talk to your doctor and see what your options are.

A broad spectrum of emotions is available to us at any time, but we often don't notice or acknowledge every feeling as it comes, largely because we wish we didn't feel certain ways. Emotions can get complicated. It's even possible to feel multiple conflicting emotions at the same time for different reasons.

Emotional awareness is not about getting rid of what you feel. It's not a hack to make your emotions go away. It's about embracing your emotions and releasing yourself from judgment about your feelings. If you like to talk, try opening up to a close friend and explaining your feelings. If not, you can journal about your emotions for a few minutes at the end of each day and see what comes out. To hope for any sort of control over your emotions, you must pay attention to them, name them, and see what patterns keep popping up.

> *"We cannot selectively numb emotions, when we numb the painful emotions, we also numb the positive emotions."*
> —*Brené Brown,* The Gifts of Imperfection[95]

SPIRITUALITY

Parenting can be a lonely road, and it can be reassuring to have something bigger than yourself to fall back on. Maybe that's God, the universe, nature, or even Oprah. Investing a chip or two in your spirituality can pay off big-time. The effect is inner peace.

> *"The transformation from being a woman to being a mother is one of beauty and power and also fear and pain. You are not in control, there are forces of the universe at work, and you are not really the star of this show. You are the medium through which another life will assert itself. During this transformation it pays to embrace uncertainty and the reality that your life is never going to be quite the same."*
> —*Zubaida Bai, Founder and CEO of Ayzh, Inc.*[96]

As a mom, you're in the trenches all the time. Motherhood can often feel like a spiritual drought, particularly if you don't practice a traditional religion. Quiet moments are nearly impossible to come by on some days. (In fact, when things are quiet around our houses, it's generally a bad sign.) A 2017 survey from the Public Religion Research Institute finds that higher levels of spirituality are strongly correlated with higher life satisfaction.[97]

---

95 Brené Brown, *The Gifts of Imperfection: Let Go of Who You Think You're Supposed To Be and Embrace Who You Are* (Center City, MN: Hazelden, 2010).
96 Zubaida Bai, "Spirituality in Motherhood and Leadership," Thrive Global, September 14, 2018, https://thriveglobal.com/stories/spirituality-in-motherhood-and-leadership/.
97 Daniel José Camacho, "Why is spirituality correlated with life satisfaction?" *The Guardian*, November 12, 2017, https://www.theguardian.com/commentisfree/2017/nov/12/spirituality-life-satisfaction-prri-study.

CHAPTER 12

Let's Get Going

"Self-care is acknowledging your self-worth, acknowledging your value to yourself. Acknowledging first to self, and then your value that you have to the people around you. Then self-care is your responsibility to your future. It's so much bigger than [getting your] nails done. It's so much bigger than a massage. Though those are nice. Self-care is saying, "I want to be responsible for my future." Meaning: "I want to give my body, give my mind, give myself, what I need so that I'm playing the long game." Self-care is recognizing this is not a sprint...this life is a marathon! Your job is to identify and have the courage and the tenacity and the resiliency to own your purpose. Your body's job is to get you there."

—*Lisa Nichols*, motivational speaker[100]

Now you know about the five main areas of life satisfaction, and you have all the tools you need to go out into the world and immediately start finding more fulfillment in every area of your life. But when? And how?

Be smart about making changes. It's never a good idea to try and change too many aspects of your life all at once. It doesn't end well. It lasts for about two days, and then you'll start to feel overwhelmed, get burnt-out,

---

100   "979 Lisa Nichols: How to Find Your Life's Purpose and Embrace Your Imperfections," *The School of Greatness with Lewis Howes* podcast, October 12, 2020, https://american-podcasts.com/podcast/the-school-of-greatness-with-lewis-howes/979-lisa-nichols-how-to-find-your-life-s-purpose-a.

think *to hell with all of this,* and eventually go right back to how you were before. Taking on too much at once is a recipe for certain disasters, especially if you have little ones who are constantly demanding your attention and all your brain power. The distractions are many and adding more things to think about can result in extra stress—and *nobody* needs that.

We recommend a gradual and steady approach to this whole changing-your-life thing. The first step is just to bring a greater level of consciousness to everything you're already doing. We're big on research, statistics, and data (if you couldn't tell), so we advocate spending some time documenting your current habits in these five areas and measuring how things are working for you. In the research world we call this establishing a baseline. If you skip this phase and just start making changes, it won't work because you won't be able to tell how well your changes are working.

This might not sound good, but it's actually great news because it means you don't have to make any hard changes just yet. The first step is easy. You're going to start by measuring your current baseline behaviors.

To get started, create a table or download the free template from our website www.happymomhappykid.com and print it out.

It looks like this:

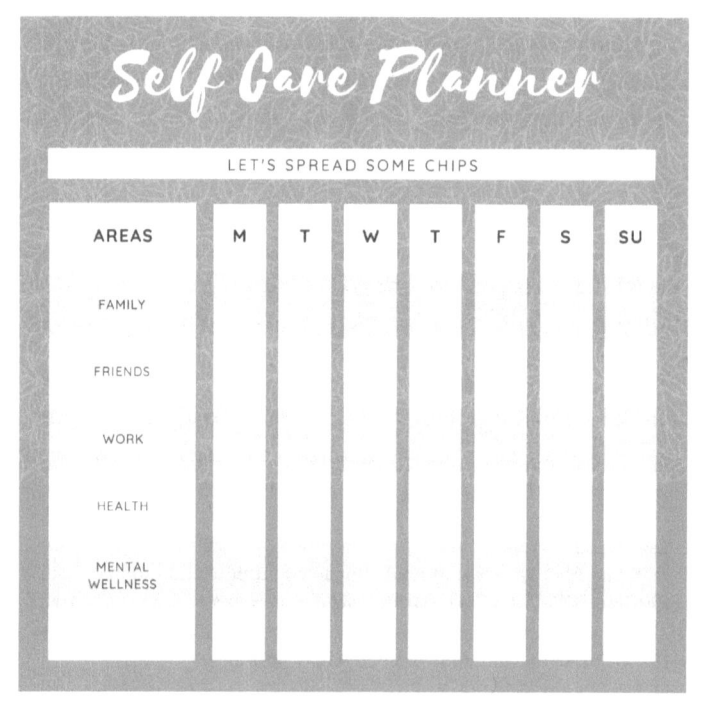

Self Care Planner

LET'S SPREAD SOME CHIPS

AREAS	M	T	W	T	F	S	SU
FAMILY							
FRIENDS							
WORK							
HEALTH							
MENTAL WELLNESS							

The idea is to place an X on each column where you've invested some chips on that particular day. For example, on a regular Monday maybe you wake the kids up, feed them, take them to school, hit the supermarket, return home, unload the groceries, get the house in order, maybe do some work, eat lunch, pick up the kids from school, take them to after-school activities, supervise homework, say hello to your fellow breeder (husband or partner), and cook and serve dinner, the end.

Consider starting to move those chips around to other areas you don't normally pay attention to. You may be doing something in these other areas anyway, but you're not focusing on them. So maybe on this Monday you will choose to do some exercise. You will still be going to Trader Joe's as scheduled, but maybe you will consciously say something nice to the lady waiting in line behind you. Instead of sitting at your computer, maybe stand for a while and then do some sit-ups. Don't overdo it; just try 10 sit-ups and then keep on working. We are talking *little stuff* here. And once you do it, you can mark it on your chart. Yay! The idea is that at the end of the week, you will be able to look back and see that you spread some chips around.

Remember, this is about looking deep inside yourself and taking some time to figure out what truly fulfills and inspires you, along with what you really need more of in your life. This isn't an opportunity to grade yourself and judge yourself for "doing it wrong." This is about taking a bit more control of your life. It's about looking closely at who you are and what version of yourself you would like to see.

Once you've monitored yourself like this for 30 days, you'll have some nice data to look through. At the end of the month, spend a couple minutes analyzing your results. Specifically, look for any patterns that jump out at you. What were you doing on the days where you felt the best? How about the days where you felt the worst? Are there any categories that you never spread any chips to? Why do you think that might be?

Based on your assessment of what's working and what's not working, make a plan for one thing you want to try doing differently during the next 30 days. The key here is to try just *one thing* at a time. This is important for a couple of reasons. First, as we mentioned before, if you try to change too many things at once, you'll burn out, feel terrible about yourself, and give up. Also, if you change more than one thing and find an improvement during the next month, you can't be sure which of your changes caused the

You just took the first step toward walking through matrescence, reclaiming control of your mom identity, solving your Rubik's Cube, and reshaping your life in a more rewarding and fulfilling way. When you implement the tools you've learned in this book, your family will benefit, your spouse will benefit, and the *world* will benefit from you sharing more of yourself through your work. But, most importantly, you will benefit from being able to live your new happier and more fulfilling life.

Remember, it all starts with you.

If this book was helpful, join our community at www.happymomhappykid.com or @happymombook and share this book with another mom in your life!

Made in United States
Troutdale, OR
07/03/2024